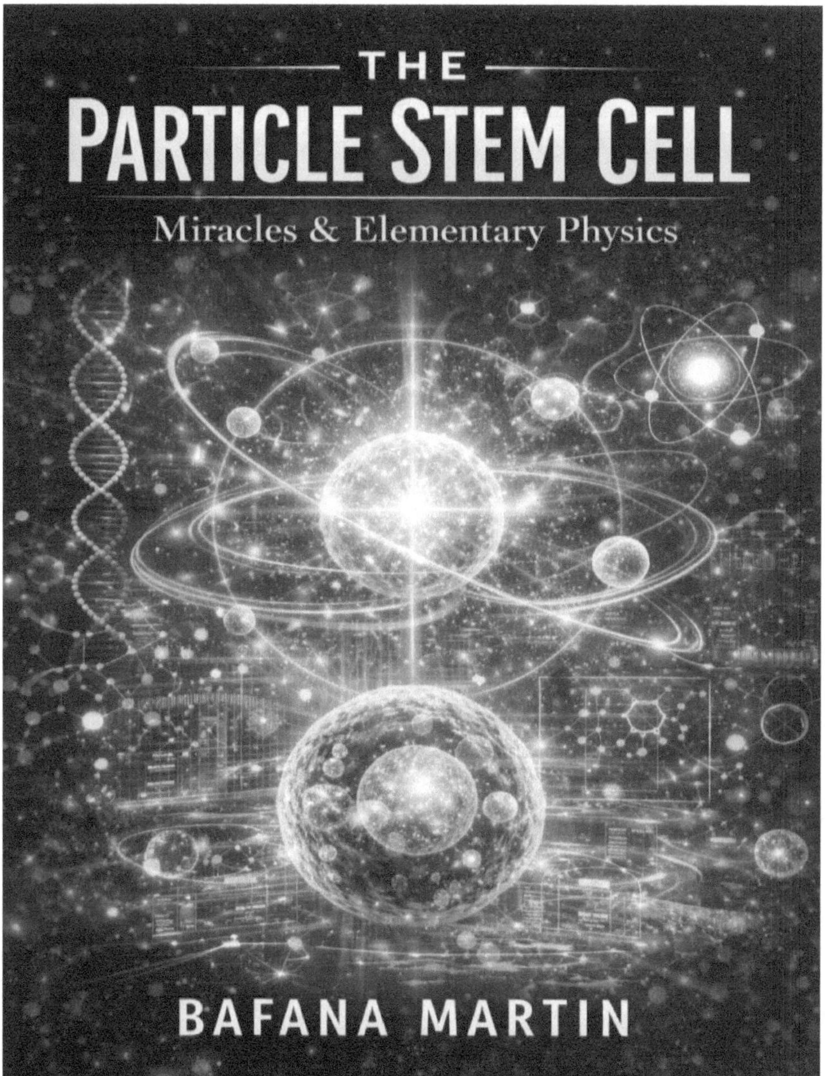
THE
PARTICLE STEM CELL
Miracles & Elementary Physics
BAFANA MARTIN

THE PARTICLE STEM CELL: MIRACLES & ELEMENTARY PHYSICS

First edition. February 26, 2026.

ISBN: 979-8233669521

Written by Bafana Martin.

THE PARTICLE STEM CELL

Miracles & Elementary Physics

By Bafana Martin

PROLOGUE

Before Differentiation

Before there were atoms, there was symmetry. Before there were stars, there were fluctuations. Before there were cells, organs, languages, and civilizations, there was undifferentiated potential — a state not of emptiness, but of infinite capacity waiting for constraint. Modern physics calls it quantum vacuum. Geometry calls it origin. Theology calls it beginning. Biology calls it stem.

Humanity has always been fascinated by miracles — by sudden restoration, unexpected manifestation, impossible reversals of decay. A blind eye opened. A limb restored. Bread multiplied. Matter appearing where none existed before. For centuries such events were placed outside natural law, beyond the reach of mechanism, sealed in sacred mystery. But what if the miraculous was never outside law? What if it was an activation of deeper law?

This book begins not with magic, but with structure. The stem cell in biology contains within it the potential to become muscle, neuron, blood, retina. It is undifferentiated yet not undefined. It is possibility under regulation. In physics, unified quantum fields contain within them the potential to differentiate into particles — electrons, quarks, photons — under symmetry breaking. Geometry reveals that from a single point, infinite lines may extend. Number reveals that from zero, infinite magnitudes unfold.

The pattern repeats across scale.

Unity precedes multiplicity.

Convergence precedes divergence.

Undifferentiated potential precedes identity.

The central question of this work is simple yet destabilizing: if differentiation governs the architecture of reality at every level, is there a foundational "stem" beneath matter itself? And if so, what would it mean to understand it? To interact with it? To specify it?

We will descend through biology into physics, through geometry into number, through alchemy into engineering, through network into atmosphere. We will explore the possibility of an elemental stem state — a transitional threshold between unified symmetry and atomic identity. We will consider what it means for matter to obey geometric instruction. We will confront the moral weight of manufacturing life.

This is not a rejection of science. It is a deepening of it. Nor is it a dismissal of miracle. It is a reinterpretation.

If matter is structured possibility, then the miraculous may not be violation — it may be precision beyond current access.

Before there was differentiation, there was potential. And potential, once understood, is never neutral. It is invitation.

This book begins at the edge of that invitation.

Table of Contents

PROLOGUE

The Undifferentiated Beginning
PART I — THE BIOLOGICAL STEM CELL (Established Science)

1. The Cell That Is Not Yet
2. Totipotent, Pluripotent, Multipotent
3. Differentiation: How Identity Forms
4. Stem Cells in Nature
5. Regeneration in Modern Medicine
6. Induced Pluripotency and Cellular Reprogramming
7. The Limits of Biological Regeneration

(This section is scientifically responsible and grounded.)

PART II — MIRACLES REEXAMINED (Speculative Biology)

1. The Blind Who Saw
2. Instant Tissue Reconstruction
3. The Acceleration Hypothesis
4. Time Compression in Living Systems
5. Matter Rearrangement vs Matter Regeneration
6. Are Miracles Violations of Nature?

(Here speculation begins, but framed as hypothesis.)

PART III — FROM CELLS TO PARTICLES (Bridging Science & Theory)

PART VII — ETHICS, FAITH, AND CREATION

EPILOGUE

Return to the Undifferentiated

Chapter 1

The Cell That Is Not Yet

Dr. Myles Darwin began every semester the same way: with an image. Projected behind him in soft fluorescence was a single human embryonic stem cell, magnified beyond natural perception, suspended in luminous stillness. It did not look extraordinary. It was round, almost plain, its membrane gently defined, its nucleus centered like a quiet star in cytoplasmic space. Yet Myles always lingered before speaking, because he knew what most of the room did not yet feel — that this unassuming structure represented one of the most radical realities in all of biology.

A stem cell is defined by two properties: it can self-renew, and it can differentiate. It can replicate itself without losing its state, and it can transform into specialized cell types that compose the human body. But those definitions, though precise, fail to capture the strangeness of what the cell truly is. It is not muscle, yet it can become muscle. It is not retina, yet it can become retina. It is not heart tissue, yet it can one day pulse as cardiac muscle. Within it lies the full genetic blueprint of an organism, but its identity has not yet been selected. It exists in a state of biological suspension — a readiness without commitment.

Inside its nucleus, DNA coils and folds in dynamic patterns. Genes are neither fully active nor permanently silent. Regulatory proteins hover in delicate balance. Molecular signals determine which sections of the genome will be expressed and which will remain quiet. Nothing is missing. Nothing needs to be added. Differentiation does not introduce new information into the cell; it selectively activates what is already present. Identity, then, is not a matter of construction from nothing — it is a matter of controlled revelation.

In the earliest stages of human development, after fertilization, the zygote divides into identical daughter cells. For a brief and astonishing window of time, each of those cells is totipotent — capable of forming an entire organism, including supporting structures like the placenta. This is the highest form of biological potential. Soon after, cells narrow into pluripotency, still capable of becoming nearly every tissue type, though no longer able to independently generate a full organism. As development continues, potential narrows further into multipotent states, where stem cells are restricted to particular lineages — blood-forming stem cells in bone marrow, neural stem cells in the brain, mesenchymal stem cells in connective tissues. Each narrowing is a step away from total possibility and a step toward defined function.

For much of modern biology, differentiation was considered irreversible. Once a skin cell became a skin cell, it remained so. Specialization was thought to be permanent. That belief held firm until the early twenty-first century, when scientists demonstrated that mature adult cells could be reprogrammed back into pluripotent states through the introduction of specific transcription factors. Identity, it turned out, was not locked. It was regulated. A skin cell could be rewound into a stem-like state. Memory could be erased. Differentiation could be reversed.

This discovery unsettled Myles more than he admitted publicly. In the laboratory upstairs from his lecture hall, he worked with induced pluripotent stem cells under sterile conditions, watching as researchers guided them toward specialized fates. Under precise chemical signaling, clusters of undifferentiated cells began to organize into beating cardiac tissue. Others formed neural structures that pulsed faintly with electrical activity. In controlled environments, primitive organoids developed — miniature livers, early retinal formations, intestinal models. Structures that did not exist days earlier emerged from clusters of cells that previously had no assigned role.

The transformation was not mystical. It was methodical. Signaling pathways activated in sequence. Genes turned on and off in carefully orchestrated cascades. Differentiation unfolded along timelines governed by molecular interaction and energy availability. Biological systems respected order. Regeneration required time.

In nature, regeneration appears in fragments. Salamanders regrow limbs. Human livers regenerate partial mass. Skin heals. Blood replenishes daily from hematopoietic stem cells residing in bone marrow niches. Even in adulthood, stem cells remain embedded within tissues, maintaining and repairing the body quietly. Yet the limits are evident. Humans cannot regrow severed limbs. Damaged optic nerves rarely repair themselves fully. Spinal cord injuries remain largely irreversible. The potential exists — but it is constrained.

Myles often found himself staring longer than necessary at the microscope display. What disturbed him was not the success of regeneration but the principle beneath it. A cell that is not yet something can become almost anything. Specialization is not the origin; it is the result. Beneath every differentiated structure lies an earlier state of undivided possibility.

He considered the hierarchy as he often did when the laboratory emptied at night. Tissues are made of cells. Cells are made of molecules. Molecules are composed of atoms. Atoms consist of elementary particles. Biology is layered upon chemistry, chemistry upon physics. If differentiation defines identity at the cellular level, what defines identity at the particle level? Does specialization begin with gene activation — or does it begin deeper, where matter itself emerges?

He did not yet voice this question to colleagues. In the university, he remained grounded in established science. He spoke of pluripotency, transcription factors, epigenetics, regenerative medicine. He emphasized the rigor of experimentation and the constraints of biological time. But privately, he sensed a pattern repeating across scales. Unity becoming multiplicity. Undifferentiated states collapsing into defined forms.

The stem cell, in its quiet spherical simplicity, was not merely a medical instrument. It was a clue. A living demonstration that identity is conditional. That form is selected, not fundamental. That beneath specialization lies a state of undivided potential.

The lecture hall would empty. The projector would dim. But the image of the undifferentiated cell would linger in his thoughts. Not muscle. Not neuron. Not retina. Only potential. A biological beginning that suggested something more universal — that perhaps differentiation itself is a law of reality, repeating from life to matter to structure.

If life begins with a cell that is not yet defined, Myles wondered in the silence of the laboratory, where does matter begin?

The semester had just begun.

Chapter 2

Totipotent, Pluripotent, Multipotent

Dr. Myles Darwin did not believe in wasting definitions. Words, like cells, carried gradients of meaning, and nowhere was this more evident than in the language of potency. Totipotent. Pluripotent. Multipotent. To his students, they were vocabulary terms for an exam. To Myles, they were stages of narrowing infinity.

He began the next lecture without dimming the lights. Instead of a single cell, the screen displayed a sequence — fertilization, division, compaction. A human zygote dividing into two cells, then four, then eight, then sixteen, forming a morula before hollowing into a blastocyst. The images were clinical, textbook-perfect. Yet beneath the diagrams lay something profound: in those earliest divisions, each cell retained the potential to generate an entire organism. Not just tissues. Not just organs. The entire body plan, including the placenta and extraembryonic membranes necessary to sustain life.

That is totipotency.

Totipotent cells exist only briefly in natural development. They represent the highest biological latitude — the ability to form every structure required for a complete organism. There is no specialization yet. No cellular destiny chosen. At this stage, division does not reduce possibility. Each daughter cell remains as capable as the original.

Myles would pause here, letting the gravity of it settle. Imagine, he would say, that every cell in your body once existed in a state where it could have become you entirely. That degree of potential is almost inconceivable. And yet it is routine in early embryogenesis.

But totipotency does not last.

Within days, differentiation begins to carve boundaries. Cells on the outer layer of the blastocyst commit to becoming trophoblasts, forming the placenta. Cells within the inner cell mass narrow into pluripotency — still capable of generating nearly every cell type in the body, but no longer able to independently form the full organism with its supporting structures.

Pluripotent cells are extraordinary, but they are no longer absolute.

From them arise the three germ layers: ectoderm, mesoderm, endoderm. The ectoderm will produce neural tissue and skin. The mesoderm will give rise to muscle, bone, blood, and connective tissue. The endoderm will form internal organs such as the liver, pancreas, and lungs. The narrowing begins not with loss of information, but with selective gene activation.

This was always the part that intrigued Myles most deeply. Nothing is subtracted from the genome during differentiation. The DNA remains intact. What changes is expression. Epigenetic markers — methyl groups, histone modifications — alter accessibility. Regulatory proteins open some chapters of the genetic library and close others. The same genetic code exists in a neuron and in a liver cell. What differs is which sections are read.

Identity, then, is a pattern of activation.

As development progresses, pluripotency yields to multipotency. Stem cells become lineage-restricted. Hematopoietic stem cells in the bone marrow produce various blood cells — red blood cells, white blood cells, platelets — but they cannot form neurons. Neural stem cells can generate neurons and glial cells but cannot produce cardiac muscle. Each step forward reduces potential while increasing functional precision.

Multipotency is specialization's final gateway.

Myles would often draw a branching diagram on the board — a tree of differentiation. At the top, a single totipotent origin. Beneath it, branching pathways representing pluripotency, then further branching into multipotent lineages, then finally into fully differentiated cells at the leaves. The tree metaphor was biologically useful but philosophically incomplete. It suggested inevitability, a linear descent into specialization.

But Myles knew something the tree did not illustrate: reversibility.

In the laboratory, induced pluripotent stem cells defied the rigidity of that tree. Through the introduction of specific transcription factors — most famously Oct4, Sox2, Klf4, and c-Myc — differentiated adult cells could be reprogrammed back into pluripotent states. The leaves of the tree could climb back toward the trunk.

This discovery disturbed older assumptions about cellular fate. If identity could be erased and rewritten, then specialization was not destiny — it was regulation. Potency was not lost; it was suppressed.

There was something almost unsettling about that realization. Beneath every differentiated cell in the human body lay a history of greater possibility. Beneath every neuron firing across synapses, there once existed a state in which that cell could have become anything else.

Possibility precedes function.

Even in adulthood, multipotent stem cells persist quietly within tissues. Hematopoietic stem cells replenish blood daily. Intestinal stem cells regenerate the lining of the gut. Epidermal stem cells repair the skin. These cells exist in niches — microenvironments that maintain their potency while preventing uncontrolled differentiation. Signals from surrounding tissues regulate their behavior. Remove them from their niche, and they may lose their identity or differentiate unpredictably.

Context shapes potential.

Myles found himself increasingly drawn to that principle. Potency is not merely an intrinsic property; it is relational. It depends on environment, signaling, constraints. A stem cell's identity is not fixed internally; it is negotiated externally.

In the private lab, he once observed a cluster of pluripotent stem cells forming embryoid bodies — spherical aggregates that spontaneously began organizing into mixed tissue types. Even without precise direction, they displayed an inherent tendency toward structured complexity. It was as though possibility carried an internal bias toward order.

But biological potency has boundaries. Totipotency fades rapidly. Pluripotency is restricted to early development or laboratory reprogramming. Multipotency is lineage-bound. There is no known natural mechanism in humans that allows full systemic regeneration. Evolution optimized survival, not total recoverability.

Why, Myles often wondered, would life encode such immense potential only to narrow it so drastically?

Energy constraints? Developmental stability? Protection against uncontrolled growth?

Cancer, after all, represents a pathological form of potency — cells dividing without regulation, differentiation failing to complete. Unchecked potential becomes destructive. Differentiation, then, is not merely limitation. It is protection.

Still, the hierarchy lingered in his mind.

Totipotent — total possibility.

Pluripotent — broad possibility.

Multipotent — restricted possibility.

Differentiated — functional identity.

Each step is a collapse of options into specificity.

The pattern felt familiar beyond biology.

In quiet moments after class, Myles would sit alone in his office and sketch again — not trees this time, but concentric narrowing circles. A center of undifferentiated potential expanding outward into increasingly defined forms. The stem cell was not simply a biological entity. It was an archetype.

An origin that contains multiplicity within unity.

And once again, as the semester deepened and research upstairs continued under sterile lighting, the same question pressed against the boundaries of his thoughts.

If biological identity narrows from totipotency into specialization...

Does matter itself follow a similar gradient?

Are elementary particles already specialized forms of something more fundamental?

Is there a deeper totipotent layer of reality — an undifferentiated substrate from which quarks, electrons, and bosons emerge as differentiated states?

He did not yet speak of such things beyond encrypted notes.

For now, he taught the hierarchy faithfully. He explained potency in its proper biological context. He emphasized regulatory pathways and developmental constraints. He cautioned against overstating regenerative potential.

But inwardly, he sensed the pattern extending beyond embryology.

Totipotent. Pluripotent. Multipotent.

Each term described not merely a biological condition, but a law of narrowing possibility.

And if that law repeated across scales — from life to matter — then the stem cell was not just a medical phenomenon.

It was a clue to the architecture of differentiation itself.

The narrowing had begun.

Chapter 3

Differentiation: How Identity Forms

If potency is possibility, differentiation is decision.

Dr. Myles Darwin opened the third week of lectures with a simple statement written across the board: **Identity is regulated.** He let the words remain there without explanation, allowing curiosity to build before unraveling the biological machinery beneath them. Because differentiation, despite its apparent elegance, is not mystical. It is molecular. It is governed by gradients, thresholds, chemical affinities, and timed cascades of gene expression.

A stem cell does not wake up and choose to become a neuron.

It is instructed.

In early embryonic development, cells exist within chemical landscapes known as morphogen gradients. These gradients consist of signaling molecules distributed unevenly across developing tissue. The concentration of these molecules determines gene activation patterns. A slight difference in position within the embryo exposes a cell to different signals, and that difference alters its developmental path. Two genetically identical cells, separated by mere micrometers, may commit to entirely different destinies.

Location becomes instruction.

Signals bind to receptors on the cell membrane. Pathways activate within the cytoplasm. Transcription factors travel into the nucleus and unlock specific sections of DNA. Some genes turn on; others are silenced. Chromatin remodels. Epigenetic markers are placed or removed. Over time, these small regulatory shifts stabilize into identity. What begins as reversible becomes reinforced. The neuron remains a neuron because its gene expression pattern becomes self-maintaining.

Differentiation is not a single event. It is a cascade.

One gene activates another. One protein suppresses a third. Feedback loops stabilize the emerging state. By the time a stem cell has matured into a specialized cell type, its internal network of regulatory interactions sustains its identity without continuous external prompting. The system becomes self-referential.

This is how muscle contracts, how neurons transmit signals, how hepatocytes detoxify blood. Each cell performs its function because differentiation configured its internal machinery for that purpose.

But Myles found something profoundly revealing in this process: differentiation does not destroy potential — it restricts access to it.

The genome remains complete. Every cell retains the same DNA sequence inherited at fertilization. The difference between a retinal cell and a cardiac cell is not the presence or absence of genetic information, but which segments are accessible. Epigenetic modifications alter chromatin structure, wrapping some genes tightly and leaving others open for transcription. The cell's identity becomes a pattern of accessibility.

In this sense, specialization is selective blindness.

A neuron does not lack the genes required to become bone; it simply cannot access them.

This realization unsettled simplistic views of identity. If differentiation is governed by regulation rather than subtraction, then in theory, identity is reversible. The discovery of induced pluripotent stem cells proved exactly that. By introducing a small set of transcription factors, scientists reactivated dormant gene networks and erased epigenetic marks. A skin cell could be returned to a pluripotent state. Identity could be dismantled.

In the private laboratory, Myles had watched this reversal occur. Fibroblasts harvested from adult tissue were exposed to carefully calibrated genetic interventions. Days passed with little visible change. Then colonies began to emerge — compact clusters resembling embryonic stem cells. Under analysis, they expressed pluripotency markers. The differentiated had become undifferentiated.

Reversal did not violate biology.

It revealed flexibility.

And yet, there were boundaries. Reprogramming was inefficient. It carried risks, including tumor formation. The cell's regulatory networks resisted destabilization. Differentiation, once stabilized, preferred to remain stable.

Why would biology resist returning to potency?

Because potency without control becomes chaos.

Cancer is, in many ways, a failure of differentiation regulation. Cells revert to proliferative states, dividing without proper specialization. They regain aspects of stem-like behavior but lack the signaling discipline required for organized development. Potential divorced from structure becomes destructive.

Thus, differentiation is both creative and protective.

It allows complexity to emerge while preventing uncontrolled expansion.

Myles often described differentiation as a narrowing funnel. At the wide top lies maximum potential. As development proceeds, pathways diverge and narrow. By the time cells reach terminal differentiation, the funnel has become a thin channel. Reversing direction requires immense intervention.

Yet beneath the complexity of signaling networks and epigenetic modification, a deeper pattern emerged. Differentiation is essentially the collapse of many possible states into one stable configuration. At any given moment, a stem cell could theoretically activate multiple developmental pathways. External signals bias the probabilities until one pathway dominates. Once stabilized, that pathway defines identity.

Probability becomes structure.

Myles could not ignore how closely this resembled another domain he rarely discussed openly in lectures: quantum mechanics. At the quantum level, particles are described not as fixed entities but as probability distributions. Only upon measurement or interaction does a system collapse into a defined state. Before observation, multiple outcomes coexist as potentialities.

He never made the comparison in class. The analogy was too speculative, too easily misunderstood. But privately, the parallel disturbed him.

In biology, differentiation collapses potential into form. In physics, observation collapses probability into particle state. In both cases, the undifferentiated precedes the defined.

He would stand alone in the underground facility late at night, reviewing cellular imaging data alongside particle interaction models projected on adjacent screens. Two fields of study, separated by scale, yet whispering the same principle.

Identity is not primary.

It is selected.

If differentiation in cells depends on environmental cues, could particle identity depend on deeper field interactions? If cellular specialization emerges from gene regulation, could particle properties emerge from a more fundamental regulatory substrate?

He considered the Higgs field — the mechanism by which particles acquire mass. In simplified terms, particles interact with a field permeating space. The degree of interaction determines mass. Mass is not inherent; it is relational.

Interaction defines property.

The pattern repeated.

Cells interact with signaling environments and acquire identity. Particles interact with fields and acquire mass. Structure emerges through relationship.

The more Myles examined differentiation, the less it appeared confined to biology. It looked like a universal strategy: begin undifferentiated, introduce constraints, stabilize identity.

He returned often to the stem cell under fluorescence. It did not look extraordinary. But within its quiet spherical form lay a dynamic equilibrium of possibility. It was a system balanced at the edge of commitment.

What determines the moment of commitment?

What defines the tipping point where potential narrows into permanence?

These were not purely biological questions. They were structural questions about reality itself.

As the lecture concluded that afternoon, students filed out discussing signaling pathways and epigenetic markers. Myles erased the board slowly, leaving only the original statement visible for a moment longer before wiping it clean:

Identity is regulated.

The words lingered in his thoughts long after the classroom emptied.

If identity at the cellular level forms through regulated collapse of potential...

What regulates the identity of matter?

And what lies beneath the first act of differentiation — beneath the first collapse into form?

The pattern was growing clearer. Differentiation is not an anomaly of life.

It is a law. And laws, once recognized, rarely remain confined to a single scale.

Chapter 4

Stem Cells in Nature

If differentiation revealed how identity forms, nature revealed why it must.

Dr. Myles Darwin shifted the focus of his lectures from the laboratory to the wild, from sterile dishes to living organisms that carried regenerative abilities far beyond those of humans. It was one thing to study stem cells under microscopes and controlled culture conditions. It was another to observe how life itself deployed them in survival.

Nature, he reminded his students, does not waste potential.

In certain species of salamander, an amputated limb does not scar over permanently. Instead, cells at the injury site undergo a remarkable transformation. Mature muscle, cartilage, and skin cells near the wound dedifferentiate — partially reverting toward a more stem-like state. A structure known as a blastema forms, composed of proliferating progenitor cells. Over weeks, guided by positional memory and signaling gradients, the lost limb regrows, complete with bone, muscle, nerves, and vasculature.

It is not a random regrowth.

It is organized reconstruction.

The blastema behaves like an orchestrated resurgence of potency. Differentiated cells loosen their identity just enough to re-enter a regenerative program. Signals reestablish developmental instructions. Tissue reconstructs itself in correct proportion.

The salamander does not panic at loss.

It reorganizes.

In zebrafish, damaged heart tissue can regenerate efficiently. In planarian flatworms, regeneration borders on astonishing. A single fragment can regrow an entire organism. These organisms possess abundant pluripotent stem cells, distributed throughout their bodies, capable of rebuilding complex systems after injury.

Why, Myles would ask quietly in class, did evolution grant some species near-total regenerative capacity while limiting humans so severely?

Humans can regenerate skin, blood, and liver tissue to a degree. The liver, in particular, demonstrates significant regenerative ability, restoring mass after partial removal. Hematopoietic stem cells replenish blood continuously. The intestinal lining renews itself every few days. Yet beyond these systems, regeneration stalls. Severed limbs do not return. Spinal cords rarely repair completely. Retinal tissue does not spontaneously reconstruct.

Some biologists argue that extensive regenerative capacity may trade off with cancer risk. Cells that can easily revert to proliferative states are more vulnerable to uncontrolled growth. Evolution may have constrained human regenerative potential to protect systemic stability.

Constraint as survival strategy.

Myles found that idea compelling but incomplete. If evolution balanced regeneration and stability, then potency must always be paired with regulation. Regeneration requires a choreography of signals, growth factors, spatial cues, and immune modulation. Without tight coordination, tissue growth devolves into chaos.

Even in regenerative species, differentiation follows order. Cells do not randomly become tissue. They follow positional information encoded in gradients and structural memory. The blastema does not forget where the elbow once was.

There is memory within regeneration.

Molecular memory.

Structural memory.

Pattern memory.

This concept fascinated Myles more deeply than he admitted. The idea that tissue could remember its form suggested that differentiation was not only activation of genes, but restoration of pattern. If regeneration replays development in compressed form, then somewhere within the organism lies a template of identity.

Not merely genetic.

But spatial.

He stood in the private lab late one evening reviewing time-lapse imaging of regenerating zebrafish tissue while across another screen particle simulations ran silently. Two domains separated by scale yet echoing similar behavior: systems destabilized and then reorganized according to underlying fields of instruction.

He began to suspect that regeneration was less about rebuilding matter and more about reactivating pattern.

If a salamander regrows a limb, it does not import new matter from outside reality. It reorganizes what exists according to encoded instructions. Cells proliferate, differentiate, and integrate along axes defined by morphogen gradients and positional signals.

Matter rearranges into pre-existing blueprint.

Could miracles, if they occurred, follow a similar principle? Could rapid regeneration represent not violation of law, but acceleration of it? If regenerative processes were compressed dramatically — if cellular proliferation, differentiation, vascular integration, and neural reconnection occurred at extraordinary speeds — would the result appear supernatural?

He never voiced these thoughts during lectures on salamanders.

Instead, he emphasized signaling pathways: Wnt, FGF, BMP. He explained blastema formation and dedifferentiation mechanisms. He described how macrophages influence regenerative outcomes, how immune response shapes healing trajectory.

But beneath the molecular detail, the pattern persisted.

Regeneration is not creation ex nihilo.

It is reactivation of latent possibility.

In humans, latent stem cells reside within niches — bone marrow, hair follicles, intestinal crypts. These niches provide microenvironments that maintain multipotent states while preventing premature differentiation. Remove a stem cell from its niche, and it may differentiate unpredictably or lose potency.

Environment stabilizes identity.

Nature does not distribute unlimited totipotency across mature organisms. Instead, it localizes potency in controlled reservoirs. The niche acts as regulator, gatekeeper, and protector.

Regeneration, then, is a controlled release of potential.

The more Myles examined regenerative biology, the more he recognized a universal constraint: undifferentiated states are powerful but unstable. They require boundaries. Totipotency fades quickly in development because unrestricted potential is energetically costly and structurally risky.

Differentiation stabilizes complexity.

And yet, somewhere deep within the architecture of life, the original potency once existed in full.

Every adult human body was once composed entirely of cells capable of becoming anything.

That fact alone unsettled him.

Because it meant that within the hierarchy of development lies a truth: specialization is secondary. The undifferentiated is primary.

He returned to his quiet office that evening and drew once more the concentric model that had begun replacing the branching tree in his notes. At the center, he wrote: **Undifferentiated Potential.** Around it, successive rings: Totipotent. Pluripotent. Multipotent. Differentiated. Tissue. Organism.

The narrowing was not just developmental.

It was architectural.

Life begins broad and becomes precise.

But the broad state is not destroyed. It is transitioned.

And if nature demonstrates that regeneration is possible through controlled reactivation of potency...

What, he wondered, would happen if the narrowing could be reversed not just in cells — but in matter itself?

The salamander regrew a limb by reactivating developmental pathways.

What if the universe itself possessed an undifferentiated state from which particles differentiate?

What if matter, like tissue, was capable of controlled regeneration from a deeper substrate?

The thought did not feel reckless.

It felt patterned.

Regeneration in nature was not an anomaly.

It was a clue.

And as the semester advanced and the private facility continued its silent research beneath the university, Myles Darwin found himself no longer asking whether regeneration was possible.

He was asking at what level it truly begins.

The narrowing of potential was not merely biological.

It might be universal.

Chapter 5

Regeneration in Modern Medicine

If nature hinted at possibility, medicine attempted to formalize it.

Dr. Myles Darwin entered the fifth week of lectures not with speculation, but with data. Clinical trials. Peer-reviewed publications. Transplant outcomes. Measured improvements in tissue repair. The students expected imagination; he gave them statistics. Because before any ascent into theory, the foundation had to be solid.

Regenerative medicine is not science fiction. It is already here — though imperfect, limited, and cautious.

Hematopoietic stem cell transplantation has been used for decades to treat blood cancers and immune disorders. Bone marrow transplants replace diseased blood-forming cells with healthy ones, effectively regenerating the patient's blood system. Skin grafts grown from epidermal stem cells restore tissue after severe burns. Corneal stem cell therapies repair damaged ocular surfaces. Mesenchymal stem cells are studied for cartilage regeneration in joint injuries. Clinical trials explore neural stem cells for spinal cord injury, though progress remains gradual.

These interventions do not regrow limbs. They do not instantly restore sight. But they demonstrate something profound: stem cells can be guided therapeutically to rebuild damaged tissue.

The promise is real.

The constraints are equally real.

One of the greatest challenges in regenerative medicine is control. Stem cells introduced into the body must differentiate into the correct cell type, integrate structurally, establish vascular connections, and avoid uncontrolled proliferation. Misguided differentiation can produce teratomas — tumors composed of mixed tissue types, a chaotic expression of pluripotency without regulation.

Potential without precision is dangerous.

In the private laboratory, Myles observed researchers coaxing induced pluripotent stem cells toward retinal lineage. Growth factors were added in precise sequences. Chemical environments shifted gradually. After weeks, organized retinal organoids began forming — primitive layered structures resembling early eye development. Under microscopes, one could see the emergence of photoreceptor precursors.

It was not sight.

But it was structure.

Elsewhere, cardiac patches grown from stem cells were being tested for repairing heart tissue damaged by myocardial infarction. Scientists attempted to bioengineer scaffolds seeded with stem cells, encouraging them to form functional muscle that could contract synchronously with existing tissue.

The progress was careful, incremental.

Regeneration in modern medicine is not instantaneous reconstruction. It is assisted development.

The body remains the primary architect.

Myles often emphasized this distinction. Regenerative medicine does not create from nothing. It stimulates or supplements the body's inherent capacity to rebuild. The cells contain the information. The therapy provides the environment.

And yet, beneath the careful clinical tone, his thoughts continued expanding.

If the limitation in modern medicine is time, what would happen if time could be compressed?

Every regenerative process — from wound healing to organoid formation — unfolds along a timeline. Stem cells proliferate. They differentiate. They migrate. They integrate. The sequence is predictable and measurable.

Time is the invisible regulator of identity.

When students asked why humans could not regrow limbs like salamanders, Myles would explain evolutionary trade-offs, immune responses, fibrosis. But internally, another question formed: what if the machinery for regeneration exists in humans, but is constrained by systemic regulation and temporal pacing?

What if the blueprint remains accessible — but the activation threshold is unreachable under ordinary conditions?

In research literature, there were occasional anomalies: children with extraordinary healing capacity, rapid tissue repair in specific contexts, experimental models showing partial regeneration under modified signaling conditions. None of it approached myth. None of it defied biology. But it hinted at elasticity.

Regenerative potential in humans is not zero.

It is limited.

And limits can be studied.

In the underground facility, beyond university oversight, Myles observed a project exploring accelerated tissue reconstruction in controlled animal models. Advanced bioelectric modulation techniques were applied to injury sites, altering membrane potentials across cells. Early results suggested that bioelectric signaling might influence regenerative outcomes more profoundly than previously understood.

Cells do not communicate only chemically.

They communicate electrically.

Voltage gradients across tissues can influence growth patterns. Bioelectric fields can act as patterning signals. Some researchers proposed that regeneration might be governed not only by genes and proteins, but by distributed electrical networks within tissues.

Pattern encoded in charge.

The idea fascinated Myles. It aligned with his growing suspicion that differentiation was not purely biochemical. It was structural and field-based.

If tissue identity is stabilized by electrical and molecular fields, then perhaps regeneration involves reestablishing those fields before matter reorganizes.

In this view, cells follow pattern fields the way iron filings follow magnetic lines.

Pattern precedes structure.

This realization deepened his unease regarding the boundary between biology and physics. Fields govern particle interactions. Bioelectric fields govern cellular behavior. Gradients guide differentiation in embryos. Charge distribution influences regeneration.

At every level, identity seemed relational — dependent on interaction within a field.

Modern medicine approaches regeneration from the bottom up: introduce cells, adjust signals, monitor outcomes. But what if regeneration could be approached from the top down — by restoring or manipulating the pattern field itself?

Would tissue then reorganize more rapidly?

Would structure emerge more efficiently?

He did not present such questions during formal lectures. Instead, he concluded the week by emphasizing caution. Stem cell therapies, he reminded his students, must be evaluated rigorously. Hype outpaces evidence. Ethical oversight is essential. Human identity and biological integrity cannot be compromised in pursuit of rapid advancement.

But alone in his office, he returned to a recurring thought.

Regeneration in medicine is limited by:

- Signaling precision
- Structural integration
- Cancer risk

• And time

Remove or compress time, and regeneration would appear miraculous.

But time compression in biology is not currently achievable at scale.

Unless — and here his thoughts grew dangerous — unless regeneration were not entirely dependent on gradual cellular proliferation.

What if matter itself could be reorganized directly according to biological blueprint?

What if instead of growing tissue slowly from stem cells, one could reconstruct it from a deeper substrate — restoring the differentiated state by accessing undifferentiated matter beneath it?

That thought marked a shift.

Modern medicine rebuilds through cell division.

But what if there exists a layer beneath cells — a more fundamental potential state — from which tissue could be regenerated instantly?

He stared at the retinal organoid imaging once more. Weeks of guided development. Structured. Predictable. Slow.

The science was remarkable.

But it was not miraculous.

And yet the existence of stem cells proved something essential: identity is not fixed. It can be reshaped.

If cells can be reprogrammed...

If tissues can be regenerated...

If patterns can be restored...

Then the concept of irreversible loss begins to fracture.

The semester continued. Research advanced incrementally. Clinical trials reported cautious optimism.

But beneath the measured progress of regenerative medicine, Dr. Myles Darwin felt the edge of a larger threshold.

Regeneration in modern medicine was not the culmination of possibility.

It was the first visible layer.

And somewhere beneath the cellular layer, beneath the molecular scaffolding, beneath even the atom — something might exist that is not yet specialized.

An undifferentiated substrate.

If accessed, it would not require weeks.

It would not require scaffolds.

It would not require gradual proliferation.

It would require only one thing:

Instruction.

And that thought no longer felt like biology alone.

It felt like the beginning of physics.

Chapter 6

Induced Pluripotency and Cellular Reprogramming

The idea that identity could be reversed had once been heresy.

For decades, biology held a quiet certainty: differentiation was terminal. A liver cell would remain a liver cell. A neuron would remain a neuron. Development was directional, irreversible, a descent from possibility into function. To suggest otherwise was to challenge the architecture of life itself.

And then the reversal happened.

Dr. Myles Darwin remembered the first time he replicated the experiment in his own laboratory. The method was precise, almost surgical in its conceptual simplicity. Adult fibroblast cells were harvested — ordinary connective tissue cells, fully differentiated, performing their quiet structural duties in the body. Into these cells, four transcription factors were introduced: Oct4, Sox2, Klf4, and c-Myc. Collectively, they would come to be known as the Yamanaka factors.

Four proteins.

Four regulatory switches.

Within weeks, colonies emerged that resembled embryonic stem cells. Genetic analysis confirmed what once seemed impossible: the fibroblasts had shed their differentiated identity. Epigenetic markers had been erased. Pluripotency genes reactivated. The cells once again expressed the molecular signature of embryonic potential.

A leaf had climbed back toward the trunk of the developmental tree.

Induced pluripotent stem cells shattered the illusion of permanent specialization. Identity, it turned out, was a stabilized state — not an absolute one. Beneath the outward structure of every differentiated cell lay regulatory circuits that could, under specific conditions, be rewired.

Reprogramming did not create new information.

It reactivated suppressed possibility.

Myles watched this process unfold under fluorescence imaging. Fibroblasts elongated and unremarkable gradually reorganized into tight, rounded colonies. Morphology shifted. Gene expression patterns transformed. Molecular markers once silent became visible.

It felt less like transformation and more like unveiling.

The genome had always contained the instructions for pluripotency. Differentiation had merely locked certain chapters away.

Unlocking them required disruption.

Reprogramming is not gentle. The introduction of transcription factors destabilizes existing regulatory networks. Cells resist reversal. Many fail. Some enter apoptosis. Others mutate. Only a fraction successfully transition into stable pluripotent states.

Identity resists erasure.

There is a biological inertia to differentiation — a momentum that preserves structure.

In lectures, Myles described the process clinically. He spoke of viral vectors delivering genetic material. He explained chromatin remodeling and methylation patterns. He outlined the risks of tumorigenesis associated with incomplete differentiation. He emphasized ethical considerations surrounding embryonic stem cell research and the importance of alternative pluripotent methods.

But internally, the implications reverberated beyond laboratory technique.

If a mature cell can be rewound...

Then differentiation is not a one-way descent.

It is a reversible modulation.

This realization altered his perception of stability. If identity at the cellular level can be undone, then specialization is not fundamental. It is contingent.

And if contingency governs biological identity...

Could it govern particle identity as well?

He stood one night in the restricted underground facility reviewing dual datasets — one from cellular reprogramming experiments, the other from quantum field simulations. On one screen, gene expression heat maps shifted as cells reverted to pluripotency. On the other, particle states emerged from fluctuations in quantum fields.

Two different languages.

One pattern.

In reprogramming, transcription factors alter the probability landscape of gene activation. They reshape which genetic states are energetically favorable. Once a threshold is crossed, the cell stabilizes in a new identity.

In quantum theory, particles are excitations of underlying fields. The field is fundamental; the particle is a localized expression. Properties emerge from interaction with that field. Mass itself arises from interaction with the Higgs field.

Fields precede particles.

Possibility precedes identity.

The parallel unsettled him.

In reprogramming, the differentiated state collapses back into a broader potential. In physics, particles collapse from probabilistic distributions into measurable states. Both involve transitions between undifferentiated and differentiated conditions.

But there was a crucial distinction.

Cellular reprogramming requires external intervention. Transcription factors must be introduced. Conditions must be altered. The system does not spontaneously reverse.

Reversal requires instruction.

Myles found himself repeating that phrase silently.

Reversal requires instruction.

If identity is regulated, then altering regulation alters identity. This was true in cells. Could it be true in matter?

What if the universe itself contains regulatory mechanisms that determine which particle states manifest? What if the "laws" of physics are stabilizing constraints similar to epigenetic locks in biology?

And what if, hypothetically, those locks could be altered?

He knew the danger of such thinking. Biology had taught him that unregulated potency produces cancer. If undifferentiated states are destabilized without precision, chaos follows. The same might apply at the particle level. Destabilizing matter's identity could yield catastrophic outcomes.

But controlled reprogramming yields pluripotency — a return to possibility without destruction.

Induced pluripotency proved that the mature is not final.

It is regulated.

In the private lab, researchers were exploring increasingly refined methods of reprogramming — chemical cocktails replacing viral vectors, bioelectric modulation influencing cell state, mechanical stiffness of substrates affecting differentiation pathways. Cells responded not only to genetic instructions, but to electrical and physical environments.

The cell is not an isolated unit.

It is a node within a field.

Signals pass through chemical gradients, electrical potentials, mechanical tensions. The cell interprets its environment and adjusts accordingly. Identity is negotiated continuously.

And that word — field — returned him again to physics.

In quantum field theory, particles are not isolated objects. They are excitations of fields that permeate space. The field exists even in vacuum. Particles are localized disturbances within that field.

What if, at a deeper level, cells themselves are localized disturbances within a biological field? What if differentiation is stabilization within that field? And what if there exists, beneath even quantum fields, a more fundamental undifferentiated substrate — a kind of universal pluripotency from which particles differentiate?

He stopped himself.

Speculation must follow evidence.

But the pattern was undeniable.

Reprogramming demonstrates that identity can be undone.

Reversal requires intervention.

Intervention requires understanding of regulatory architecture.

If the regulatory architecture of matter were understood — fully understood — could matter be reprogrammed?

The thought carried both promise and terror.

In regenerative medicine, reprogramming holds hope for replacing damaged tissue. In physics, reprogramming matter would mean reshaping reality itself.

He returned to his office late that evening and opened his encrypted notebook. On a blank page, he wrote:

If a differentiated cell can be rewound to pluripotency through regulatory intervention, could a differentiated particle be rewound to a more fundamental undifferentiated state?

He paused, then added beneath it:

What is the Yamanaka factor of matter?

The question felt absurd.

And yet, every major scientific shift begins as a question that feels absurd.

Induced pluripotency had already rewritten biology's understanding of identity. It proved that specialization is not permanent — only stabilized.

If stabilization can be altered...

Then the narrowing of possibility is not destiny.

It is control.

And somewhere beneath the differentiated particles that compose matter — beneath electrons and quarks and bosons — there might exist a deeper, undifferentiated state.

A totipotency of reality.

The semester advanced.

The research continued.

But within Dr. Myles Darwin, a reversal had already begun.

He no longer saw stem cells as isolated biological tools.

He saw them as evidence.

Evidence that identity — at every level — may be more flexible than assumed.

And flexibility, once understood, changes everything.

Chapter 7

The Limits of Biological Regeneration

By the seventh week of the semester, Dr. Myles Darwin did something he rarely did in his lectures.

He dismantled hope.

Not to discourage his students, but to discipline them.

Regenerative medicine was advancing. Stem cells were powerful. Reprogramming had reshaped biology's understanding of identity. Organoids pulsed in glass chambers. Tissue engineering labs promised revolutionary treatments. But promise is not proof. And biology, for all its elegance, obeys constraints.

There are limits.

Myles stood before the class and projected two images side by side. On the left, a regenerating salamander limb. On the right, a human amputee.

"Why," he asked quietly, "can one rebuild and the other cannot?"

The answers came predictably: evolutionary trade-offs, immune response differences, fibrosis, genetic suppression of regenerative pathways.

All correct.

But incomplete.

Human regeneration fails at scale not because the body lacks stem cells, but because the architecture of regeneration is inhibited. When a severe injury occurs in humans, the immune system responds aggressively. Inflammation rises. Scar tissue forms. Fibroblasts lay down collagen rapidly to seal wounds. This fibrosis stabilizes the injury but prevents organized regrowth. Scar tissue is biologically protective — but structurally limiting.

Protection overrides restoration.

In salamanders, the immune response is more permissive. Instead of rapid fibrosis, there is controlled dedifferentiation. Mature cells near the injury site loosen their identity, proliferate, and re-enter developmental programs. Humans, by contrast, seal and stabilize.

Evolution optimized for survival speed, not structural perfection.

Myles explained that regenerative capacity depends on multiple factors: cellular plasticity, immune modulation, bioelectric patterning, vascular support, and positional memory. Remove or distort any one of these elements, and regeneration collapses.

And then there is cancer.

The closer a system moves toward undifferentiated proliferation, the greater the risk of uncontrolled growth. Stem cells divide. Cancer cells divide. The distinction lies in regulation. Regenerative capacity requires careful orchestration. Too little, and healing fails. Too much, and tumors form.

Nature appears to have drawn a line.

Humans possess limited regenerative capacity — enough for maintenance, insufficient for complete reconstruction.

Why would life encode such extraordinary potential in early development only to suppress it so firmly in maturity?

Because stability requires narrowing.

A fully totipotent adult organism would be biologically unstable. Every injury could trigger uncontrolled dedifferentiation. Every environmental fluctuation could destabilize identity. Differentiation provides structural reliability. It anchors form.

But the existence of early potency proves something undeniable: total regenerative potential once existed.

The embryo does not scar.

The embryo reorganizes.

In early developmental stages, injuries can be repaired seamlessly. Tissue integrates without fibrosis. Structural blueprints are still fluid. The closer a system remains to undifferentiated potential, the more flexible its recovery.

Flexibility declines with specialization.

The pattern was unmistakable.

The more defined identity becomes, the harder it is to undo.

Myles returned again to the laboratory upstairs. Petri dishes glowed softly under incubator lights. In one chamber, stem cells were being directed toward neural lineages. In another, cardiac differentiation protocols ran precisely timed sequences of growth factor exposure. Weeks of careful orchestration.

Biological regeneration obeys time.

Cells must proliferate. Vessels must form. Neural networks must reconnect. Differentiation cascades must unfold in sequence. Even if all signaling pathways are optimized, regeneration remains temporal.

And time is not optional.

Without sufficient time for cellular division and integration, tissue cannot rebuild.

This is the ultimate biological constraint.

Regeneration is not instantaneous.

It is developmental replay.

Myles felt the tension tighten within him. Because if regeneration requires time, and miracles — as described in ancient accounts — appear instantaneous, then either those accounts are metaphorical, exaggerated, or misinterpreted... or they operate under mechanisms beyond standard biological pacing.

He did not speak of this tension in class.

Instead, he summarized the limits clinically:

- Scar formation inhibits large-scale regrowth.

- Cancer risk constrains unrestricted proliferation.
- Positional memory degrades with maturity.
- Bioelectric and molecular patterning is difficult to restore fully.
- Time governs all regenerative processes.

And yet.

The limits themselves pointed toward something deeper.

If regeneration is limited by regulation and time, then altering regulation or time would alter outcomes.

But altering time biologically is not currently feasible. Accelerating cell division indiscriminately would induce malignancy. Compressing developmental cascades could destabilize structure.

Unless regeneration did not depend solely on gradual proliferation.

Unless there exists a more fundamental layer of identity beneath cells — beneath molecules — where matter itself could be reorganized according to blueprint without waiting for division cycles.

He returned once more to the hierarchy:

Tissue → Cells → Molecules → Atoms → Particles.

Biological regeneration rebuilds at the cellular level upward. It relies on cells dividing and differentiating. But what if reconstruction could occur at the particle level downward?

Instead of growing tissue, what if tissue could be reassembled?

Instead of weeks of differentiation, what if identity could be reinstated by accessing undifferentiated matter beneath specialized form?

The idea hovered at the edge of plausibility and impossibility.

But stem cell biology had already demonstrated something radical: identity is not absolute. It is conditional and reversible within constraints.

The limits of biological regeneration did not extinguish possibility.

They clarified the boundary.

And boundaries are where new hypotheses are born.

Myles stood alone in the underground facility, lights dimmed, particle field simulations glowing faintly on a curved screen. He overlaid a visualization of cellular differentiation cascades beside quantum field excitations. Two systems governed by probability landscapes. Two systems stabilized by regulatory constraints.

If biological regeneration is limited by differentiation lock-in...

Then perhaps the true key to unlimited regeneration does not lie in cells.

It lies in the substrate from which cells emerge.

The semester had now established the scientific foundation. Potency exists. Differentiation regulates identity. Reprogramming can reverse specialization. Regeneration is possible but constrained.

The limits were clear.

And clarity sharpened the next question.

If biology cannot regenerate instantly because it operates within cellular constraints...

What lies beneath those constraints?

What layer of reality remains undifferentiated?

The narrowing had been studied.

Now it was time to examine what precedes it.

The course was about to shift from biology to matter itself.

Chapter 8

The Blind Who Saw

The transition began quietly.

Dr. Myles Darwin did not introduce the next lecture with a diagram or a dataset. He wrote a single sentence across the board:

What would it take to restore sight instantly?

The room remained still.

Until this point, the course had remained firmly grounded in biology — stem cell hierarchies, differentiation cascades, regenerative constraints. Now the question hovered at the edge of discomfort. Not theological. Not devotional. Structural.

He did not mention scripture.

He mentioned anatomy.

To restore sight in a person born without functional vision, multiple systems must align. Photoreceptor cells in the retina must detect light. Bipolar and ganglion cells must transmit signals. The optic nerve must relay impulses to the visual cortex. Neural circuits in the occipital lobe must interpret patterns as image. Blood vessels must nourish the tissue. Synaptic connections must be precisely organized.

Sight is not a single structure.

It is an integrated system.

In cases of degenerative retinal disease, stem cell therapy has been explored. Researchers attempt to replace damaged photoreceptors using pluripotent-derived retinal cells. But integration is complex. Transplanted cells must align with existing circuitry. Axons must extend correctly. Synapses must form accurately. Even small misalignments disrupt function.

Regeneration of sight, biologically, is a layered reconstruction.

And it is slow.

Myles described cases of corneal stem cell transplantation restoring vision in patients whose blindness resulted from surface damage. That form of restoration is medically plausible. But regeneration of optic nerves or fully reconstructed retinas remains an immense challenge.

Time again asserted itself as a constraint.

Cell proliferation requires days. Tissue integration requires weeks. Neural plasticity requires sustained adaptation. Even if the correct stem cells were introduced and guided perfectly, immediate restoration would defy current biological pacing.

Which brought him back to the question written on the board.

What would it take?

He allowed the silence to stretch before answering his own inquiry.

To restore sight instantly, one of two mechanisms would need to occur:

Either biological regeneration must operate at impossible speed — compressing weeks or months into seconds — or the necessary structures must already exist in some undifferentiated or latent state and simply require activation.

The second possibility intrigued him more.

What if blindness, in some hypothetical cases, were not absence of structure but suppression of function? What if restoration did not require construction, but reconfiguration?

Neural plasticity demonstrates that the brain can rewire itself to a degree. Sensory cortices can reorganize. Latent circuits can activate under altered conditions. But even neuroplasticity operates along time scales measurable in days, weeks, or months.

Instantaneous reconfiguration remains outside biological precedent.

Unless — and here his thoughts pressed further — unless reconstruction did not occur through cellular growth at all.

Unless matter itself reorganized.

He turned from the board and faced the students.

"If tissue could be reassembled at the particle level," he said slowly, choosing each word carefully, "then regeneration would not require cellular division."

A few students shifted uncomfortably. The statement bordered on science fiction.

He continued, grounding the speculation.

"Every retinal cell is composed of molecules. Molecules are composed of atoms. Atoms are composed of particles. If the arrangement of those particles defines structure, then altering the arrangement defines identity."

He did not claim such alteration was possible.

He asked what it would imply.

If the retinal tissue of a blind individual were reassembled from existing matter — if molecular architecture were corrected instantly — then vision would be restored without waiting for cell proliferation.

It would not be biological growth.

It would be structural reorganization.

He erased the board and wrote two phrases beneath the original question:

Biological Regeneration

Structural Reassembly

Biological regeneration relies on stem cells, differentiation, and time.

Structural reassembly would require access to a more fundamental layer of matter.

He did not mention miracles explicitly, but the tension hung in the room. Ancient accounts of instantaneous healing — the blind who saw, the lame who walked — could be interpreted metaphorically. Or exaggerated. Or symbolic.

But if taken literally, they would require a mechanism beyond known biological pacing.

The purpose of the lecture was not to validate scripture.

It was to explore mechanism.

Mechanism separates superstition from hypothesis.

In the underground facility later that evening, Myles replayed retinal imaging data while particle interaction models shimmered across the adjacent screen. If a retinal layer were destroyed and needed restoration, could matter be reorganized directly according to stored blueprint? Could positional information embedded within neural architecture guide particle reassembly?

In regenerative biology, pattern fields guide development. In physics, fields guide particle behavior. The retina forms according to gradients and spatial cues. Particles align according to field equations.

The parallel was no longer subtle.

If a salamander regrows a limb by reactivating developmental patterning...

And if human regeneration is constrained by regulatory limitations...

Then instantaneous restoration would require bypassing cellular cascades entirely.

It would require access to undifferentiated substrate.

The more he examined it, the clearer the dichotomy became.

Stem cells represent biological potential.

But biological potential is already specialized relative to particle potential.

Stem cells are multipotent or pluripotent — not fundamental. They are composed of differentiated particles arranged into molecular complexity. Even totipotent cells exist within atomic constraints.

If there exists a deeper layer — a "particle stem cell," an undifferentiated quantum substrate capable of differentiating into any known particle — then structural reassembly would not violate biology.

It would precede it.

In that framework, instantaneous restoration would not compress time.

It would bypass developmental time entirely.

He closed his eyes briefly, allowing the weight of the idea to settle.

If matter itself were programmable at the most fundamental level...

Then healing would become engineering.

The classroom had ended hours earlier. The facility was silent. Only the faint hum of computational systems filled the chamber.

He opened his encrypted journal again and wrote:

Biological stem cells regenerate through time.

A particle stem cell would regenerate through structure.

He paused.

If such a substrate exists, it would not merely restore sight.

It would redefine identity itself.

The blind who saw would not represent suspension of law.

It would represent application of deeper law.

He leaned back in his chair, staring at the overlapping projections of retinal tissue and quantum field models.

Biology narrows possibility.

Physics stabilizes form.

But beneath both may lie an undifferentiated layer — a foundational potency from which matter differentiates.

The semester had crossed a threshold.

The next step would no longer belong purely to biology.

It would require stepping into the architecture of matter itself.

And once that step was taken, there would be no returning to conventional limits.

Because if structural reassembly is possible...
Then miracles are not supernatural.
They are technical.

Chapter 9

Instant Tissue Reconstruction

The question was no longer whether regeneration was possible. The question was how fast structure could be rebuilt.

Dr. Myles Darwin stood alone in the underground facility as high-resolution simulations of cellular regeneration played across a curved wall of light. One projection displayed conventional wound healing: inflammation, clot formation, immune infiltration, fibroblast activation, collagen deposition, tissue remodeling. The sequence unfolded across days and weeks, compressed into minutes for visualization.

On the adjacent screen, he replayed embryonic development: rapid cellular divisions, coordinated differentiation, spatial patterning guided by morphogen gradients. Faster than adult healing, but still sequential. Still dependent on replication and growth.

Biology reconstructs through accumulation.

Cell by cell.

Division by division.

Time is not merely a parameter in regeneration — it is the scaffolding.

And yet, the concept that had begun forming within him no longer rested comfortably inside biological timelines.

If instantaneous tissue reconstruction were to occur — true immediate restoration of structure — it could not rely on mitosis. Cells cannot divide thousands of times in seconds without catastrophic failure. DNA replication requires enzymatic precision. Chromosomes must segregate accurately. Membranes must form. Organelles must assemble. Even accelerated biological systems obey molecular pacing.

To compress this into moments would exceed metabolic limits.

Unless reconstruction does not proceed upward from cells.

Unless it proceeds downward from structure.

He turned his attention to a separate dataset — molecular modeling of retinal architecture. Each photoreceptor cell consisted of precisely arranged proteins, lipid membranes, ion channels, cytoskeletal frameworks. The organization was not random. It was hierarchical. Proteins formed complexes. Complexes formed structures. Structures formed tissue layers.

Identity at every level was arrangement.

Molecular arrangement determines cellular function.

Atomic arrangement determines molecular behavior.

Particle configuration determines atomic properties.

If identity equals arrangement, then reconstruction equals rearrangement.

He leaned forward.

Suppose a damaged retina does not need to grow anew from stem cells. Suppose the surrounding matter — already composed of atoms and molecules — could be reorganized into correct configuration instantly. Instead of proliferating cells gradually, what if matter could be repositioned at fundamental levels according to stored blueprint?

That blueprint might exist in genetic code, bioelectric patterning, or residual structural memory within the nervous system.

The critical question became this:

What layer of matter must be accessed to enable direct reassembly?

Cells are too slow.

Molecules are more fundamental, but their rearrangement still requires energy and chemical pathways.

Atoms? Rearranging atoms demands overcoming bond energies, but perhaps in principle possible.

Particles?

At the particle level, matter becomes field excitations. Particles are not rigid building blocks; they are quantized disturbances in underlying fields. Their properties emerge from interactions.

If a deeper undifferentiated particle state exists — a substrate capable of differentiating into any particle configuration — then reconstruction could bypass molecular chemistry entirely.

Matter would not be rebuilt chemically.

It would be reinstated structurally.

He replayed retinal cross-sections on the display. Photoreceptors, bipolar cells, ganglion cells layered in delicate precision. Axons projecting toward the optic nerve. The entire structure could be described as spatial information encoded in matter.

Information defines structure.

If information is preserved — even partially — then structure could theoretically be restored.

The difficulty lies in mechanism.

How would matter reorganize without gradual assembly?

He considered bioelectric patterning once more. Research had shown that electrical fields across tissues influence growth patterns. In some experimental models, altering bioelectric gradients could induce ectopic eye formation in amphibians. Change the field, and tissue reorganizes accordingly.

The field instructs.

Cells follow.

What if matter itself responds to a more fundamental field — one capable of specifying particle arrangement directly?

He stood, pacing slowly across the dim chamber.

In quantum theory, particles are excitations of fields that permeate space. The field is primary. The particle is secondary. The vacuum itself is not empty; it is structured.

If a field can give rise to particles, could altering that field give rise to new configurations of particles?

Could localized field modulation reconstruct tissue?

He stopped.

Such control lies far beyond current technological capability.

But the theoretical framework suggested something radical:

Instant tissue reconstruction would require not acceleration of biology, but intervention at the level of matter's underlying field.

He recalled again the earlier hierarchy:

Tissue → Cells → Molecules → Atoms → Particles → Fields.

Biological regeneration operates from cells upward.

Instant reconstruction would require intervention from fields downward.

The distinction was enormous.

One pathway requires time and growth.

The other requires control and specification.

He opened a new file in his encrypted journal and typed:

Instant reconstruction is not accelerated biology.

It is field-mediated reassembly.

The words felt dangerous.

If true — even hypothetically — the implications extended beyond healing.

If tissue can be reconstructed instantly, then any matter configuration can be constructed instantly.

The difference between repair and creation collapses.

He returned to the retinal simulation and imagined reversing destruction not through growth, but through reinstatement. A blind eye restored not by weeks of differentiation, but by immediate reconfiguration of matter according to preexisting pattern.

The ancient accounts described touch.

Command.

Immediate change.

In modern terms, such change would require a field interaction capable of specifying structure directly.

He exhaled slowly.

He was no longer examining stem cells alone.

He was examining the possibility that reality itself might possess a regenerative layer deeper than biology.

If instantaneous reconstruction is possible, then matter is not static.

It is responsive.

Responsive to what?

Instruction.

And if instruction can operate at the level of fundamental fields, then matter is programmable.

He felt the threshold approaching.

Up to this point, his investigation had remained anchored in biological plausibility. Now the inquiry demanded entry into particle physics.

Because to understand reconstruction beyond time, he would have to understand how particles emerge from fields in the first place.

The next question was unavoidable.

What is an elementary particle?

And could there exist a particle that is not yet specialized?

A particle stem cell.

The term lingered in his mind like a forbidden symmetry.

Biology had taught him that undifferentiated states precede specialization.

Physics might reveal whether matter obeys the same law.

The boundary between healing and creation was thinning.

And he was about to cross it.

Chapter 10

The Acceleration Hypothesis

Dr. Myles Darwin did not begin the next lecture with theology, nor with particle fields, nor even with stem cells.

He began with time.

"Every biological process," he said quietly, "has a velocity."

He turned and projected a graph onto the screen — wound healing progression plotted against days. Inflammation peaked within hours. Proliferation followed. Collagen deposition rose gradually. Remodeling extended over weeks. The curve was unmistakable: healing unfolds sequentially.

Then he projected another — embryonic development stages plotted across weeks. Neural tube formation. Limb bud emergence. Organogenesis. Again, a timeline. Ordered. Measurable. Predictable.

Biology does not jump.

It progresses.

And yet, accounts of instantaneous healing — whether religious, mythological, or anecdotal — describe something different. No swelling. No intermediate tissue. No visible proliferation. Sight restored. Limbs strengthened. Skin cleansed.

Immediate.

Myles did not argue for their literal accuracy.

He asked a different question:

"If such events were biologically real," he said, "what would have to change?"

The room remained silent.

He wrote two phrases on the board:

Acceleration of Process

Bypass of Process

The first was simpler to imagine.

What if regeneration simply occurred faster? What if cellular division, differentiation, vascular integration, and neural rewiring were compressed into seconds instead of weeks?

He began calculating aloud.

A human retinal layer contains millions of photoreceptor cells. For regeneration to occur within seconds through standard biological proliferation, mitotic cycles would have to occur thousands of times faster than known enzymatic replication allows. DNA polymerase operates at measurable rates. Chromosome segregation requires precise spindle formation. Cytokinesis cannot occur without membrane assembly.

There are biochemical ceilings.

Accelerate cell division too much, and fidelity collapses. Mutation rates explode. Structural errors multiply. Cancer becomes inevitable.

Biology is limited not by imagination, but by chemistry.

So simple acceleration — compressing time while preserving mechanism — quickly collides with physical constraint.

He erased "Acceleration of Process" and circled the second phrase instead.

Bypass of process.

This was more radical.

If regeneration does not occur through rapid cell division, then what is being bypassed? The cascade itself.

Perhaps tissue does not need to grow.

Perhaps it needs to be restored.

He turned back to retinal diagrams projected on the screen.

A retina is not just a collection of cells. It is spatial information encoded in molecular arrangement. Photoreceptors align in precise layers. Synaptic junctions follow structured pathways. Vascular support integrates seamlessly.

What if that structure, once destroyed, could be reinstated by reestablishing pattern — not by generating new cells, but by reconfiguring existing matter?

He paused, then said something he had never spoken in a lecture hall before:

"What if time is not being compressed... but skipped?"

The hypothesis began forming clearly in his mind now.

Biological regeneration requires time because it operates at the cellular level. But if structure could be restored at a deeper level — molecular or even particle — then time-dependent proliferation would be unnecessary.

Matter would not need to grow.

It would need to reorganize.

The Acceleration Hypothesis, as he began defining it privately in his notes, did not claim that biological processes move faster. It proposed that biological intermediates are bypassed entirely.

Instead of:

Stem cell activation → proliferation → differentiation → integration

There would be:

Structural reinstatement → functional restoration

Instantaneous healing, under this framework, would not be hyper-fast biology.

It would be structural reset.

He returned again to physics in his thoughts.

At the quantum level, transitions can occur discontinuously. Electrons do not move gradually between energy states; they "jump." Phase transitions in matter — water freezing, metals becoming superconductive — occur when underlying conditions shift past thresholds.

What appears gradual at macro scale may involve discrete shifts at micro scale.

Could biological structure, under extraordinary field influence, undergo a kind of phase transition?

He began outlining the hypothesis clearly:

1. Biological tissue contains structural information embedded in molecular and bioelectric patterns.
2. Damage disrupts the arrangement but may not erase all pattern information.
3. If a deeper substrate of matter exists — an undifferentiated quantum field state — then re-specification of that field could restore prior configuration instantly.
4. The visible result would appear as accelerated regeneration, though it would actually be direct reassembly.

Acceleration would be an illusion.

Bypass would be the mechanism.

He sat later that night in the underground facility reviewing models of symmetry breaking in particle physics. When underlying field conditions shift, particles differentiate into stable configurations rapidly. The early universe did not slowly grow quarks from nothing over millennia; differentiation occurred through phase transitions as energy conditions changed.

Reality itself had once undergone instantaneous structural shifts.

If such transitions are natural at cosmological scale, could localized micro-scale field transitions reorganize matter?

The thought was dangerous.

If structural reinstatement is possible, then healing is merely one application. Destruction could occur just as easily. Rearrangement could produce any configuration.

He leaned back in his chair and closed his eyes.

The Acceleration Hypothesis does not argue that miracles violate natural law.

It argues that they operate at a deeper layer of law.

The key distinction is crucial.

If time-bound biological processes are bypassed, then the true mechanism lies beneath biology.

In that case, stem cells are not the ultimate explanation.

They are a surface expression of a deeper regenerative architecture.

The semester had now crossed from safe biology into controlled speculation.

He knew it.

The students sensed it.

And beneath the campus, the facility's particle models shimmered with increasing relevance.

If regeneration can bypass cellular time...

Then the next question is unavoidable:

What is the substrate that allows bypass?

What is the undifferentiated layer from which matter itself differentiates?

The Acceleration Hypothesis was no longer a theological question.

It was a structural one.

And answering it would require stepping fully into the architecture of elementary physics.

The boundary between healing and field theory was dissolving.

And Dr. Myles Darwin was no longer merely studying stem cells.

He was studying the speed of creation itself.

Chapter 11

Time Compression in Living Systems

The Acceleration Hypothesis raised a dangerous possibility: what appears instantaneous may not violate law — it may operate at a deeper level of it. But before Dr. Myles Darwin allowed himself to descend fully into particle speculation, he disciplined the idea with biology once more.

If process could not be skipped, could time itself be compressed?

Time in biology is not abstract. It is chemical. It is governed by reaction rates, enzyme kinetics, diffusion limits, membrane transport speeds, ATP availability, and thermodynamic constraints. Cells do not experience time as humans do. They experience it as molecular turnover.

He stood before a projection showing DNA replication. Polymerase enzymes moved along strands at defined speeds. Proofreading mechanisms corrected errors. Replication forks advanced at measurable rates. There was no room for infinite acceleration without error.

Even the fastest biological systems obey limits.

Neural transmission, for instance, occurs in milliseconds — astonishingly fast compared to wound healing. Ion channels open and close within microseconds. Action potentials propagate along axons at high velocity. Synaptic transmission releases neurotransmitters in tightly timed bursts.

But even neurons do not leap outside causality.

There is delay.

There is conduction velocity.

There is sequence.

Myles began analyzing whether any biological system demonstrated meaningful time compression. He examined embryogenesis — where massive structural complexity unfolds in weeks rather than years. He examined immune response — where billions of antibodies can be generated rapidly through clonal expansion. He examined cellular stress responses — where transcriptional shifts occur within minutes.

Acceleration exists in biology.

But acceleration is bounded.

Every increase in speed requires increased energy, increased metabolic load, increased risk of error. Compress biological time too aggressively, and systems destabilize.

He wrote on the board:

Biological Time = Chemical Reaction Speed + Energy Availability + Error Tolerance

Remove any one variable, and collapse follows.

So true time compression — compressing weeks into seconds — would require reaction speeds thousands of times greater than current biochemical ceilings. That would demand energy densities incompatible with cellular survival.

Cells would vaporize before regenerating.

Thus, biological time cannot simply be forced into acceleration without catastrophic consequence.

He returned to the salamander once more. Limb regeneration takes weeks. Even in the most regenerative species, time is required for cell migration, proliferation, differentiation, and integration.

Nature does not demonstrate instantaneous macroscopic regeneration.

Unless what appears instantaneous is actually reconfiguration at a deeper scale.

He paused on that thought.

Because time at different scales is not uniform in perception.

At quantum scales, processes occur in femtoseconds and attoseconds — time intervals so small they escape intuitive comprehension. Phase transitions at atomic levels can occur extremely rapidly compared to biological processes.

If structural reassembly occurs at particle scales, it may not require biological time at all.

He felt the idea stabilizing into clarity.

Biological systems cannot compress time beyond chemical limits.

But field-level transitions operate under different rules.

In physics, when a system crosses a critical threshold, a phase transition occurs nearly instantly relative to macro-scale observation. Superconductivity emerges when temperature drops below a critical point. Water crystallizes into ice when molecular motion slows past threshold. The transformation appears abrupt because it is governed by field conditions rather than gradual assembly.

The pattern returned again:

Field condition shift → structural change.

If living tissue is fundamentally matter organized under biological fields, then altering deeper field conditions could reorganize structure faster than cellular processes allow.

Time would not be compressed biologically.

It would be irrelevant.

The visible restoration of structure would appear instantaneous because the mechanism bypasses sequential assembly.

He paced slowly through the underground facility, reviewing layered data. One screen displayed bioelectric field mappings of developing embryos. Another displayed Higgs field interaction models. Both revealed invisible landscapes shaping visible structure.

Fields govern form.

If one could access or modulate a field deeper than molecular interaction — a substrate beneath known quantum fields — then structural reassembly might occur without violating chemistry.

Chemistry would simply obey new boundary conditions.

He stopped in front of the particle simulation array and whispered:

"Acceleration is an illusion. It is phase change."

He returned to his encrypted journal.

The Acceleration Hypothesis Refined:

Instantaneous healing is not compression of biological time.

It is a phase-level structural reinstatement governed by deeper field modulation.

He considered the implications carefully.

If true, then ancient descriptions of immediate healing would not represent suspension of law. They would represent intervention at a level beneath law as currently understood.

This did not prove such events occurred.

But it established a theoretical framework in which they would not be impossible.

The classroom had grown increasingly silent in recent weeks as his lectures deepened. Students sensed the shift from conventional biology toward boundary territory. Some were intrigued. Some unsettled. A few took furious notes, recognizing the audacity of the synthesis.

Myles did not present conclusions.

He presented architecture.

Time in living systems is constrained by chemistry.

Chemistry is constrained by atomic interaction.

Atomic interaction is governed by particle fields.

If there exists a deeper undifferentiated substrate — a pre-differentiated field state — then phase-level reconfiguration could bypass chemical time entirely.

He exhaled slowly.

The Acceleration Hypothesis was no longer about speed.

It was about depth.

And depth always reveals something unsettling:

The closer one moves toward foundational layers of reality, the less fixed structure appears.

Particles are not solid.

Fields are not static.

Symmetry can break.

Identity can emerge.

And if identity can emerge, perhaps it can also be reinstated.

He closed the simulation display and stood in darkness for a moment.

Biology had brought him to the edge.

Time compression in living systems had clarified the limits.

The next step would require entering physics without restraint.

Because if acceleration is not the answer...

Then the true question is this:

What is the undifferentiated quantum state?

And could it be accessed?

The semester had reached its inflection point.

The narrowing was complete.

Now he would descend to the root.

Chapter 12

Matter Rearrangement vs. Matter Regeneration

By the time Dr. Myles Darwin returned to the lecture hall, the tone of the course had shifted permanently.

He no longer stood only as a biologist explaining stem cell hierarchies. He stood at the threshold between regeneration and ontology — between healing and the nature of matter itself.

On the board he wrote two phrases:

Matter Rearrangement

Matter Regeneration

Then he stepped back.

"Most regenerative medicine," he began, "is rearrangement."

When a bone fractures, cells migrate. Collagen scaffolds form. Osteoblasts deposit new matrix. Blood vessels reconnect. The atoms that rebuild the bone come from nutrients already circulating in the body. Nothing is created from nothing. Matter is redistributed and reorganized.

Rearrangement obeys conservation.

In chemical reactions, bonds break and reform. Molecules recombine. Atoms are neither created nor destroyed. They are repositioned within structural frameworks.

Even stem cell differentiation is rearrangement. Gene expression shifts. Proteins assemble differently. Cytoskeletal structures reorganize. But the underlying atomic inventory remains constant.

Rearrangement is lawful and measurable.

Regeneration, as currently understood, is complex rearrangement guided by biological instruction.

But what, he asked quietly, would true regeneration mean?

If a blind eye lacked functional retinal tissue — if cells were absent rather than damaged — then rearrangement of existing tissue might be insufficient. There would need to be an influx of matter to reconstruct what was missing.

Where would that matter originate?

In biological regeneration, it comes from the bloodstream — from nutrients and cellular proliferation. But that process requires time.

Instantaneous restoration would require either instantaneous importation of matter or transformation of surrounding matter into required tissue.

Which raises an unsettling distinction.

Is healing the rearrangement of existing matter?

Or is it regeneration from a deeper substrate?

He turned to the projection screen and displayed a molecular model of retinal photoreceptor proteins. Rhodopsin molecules embedded in lipid membranes. Ion channels aligned precisely. Structural arrangement defined function.

"Function," he said slowly, "is arrangement."

If the arrangement can be restored, function returns.

But the restoration of arrangement requires control at some level of matter.

He began analyzing the problem systematically.

If a structure is destroyed, its constituent atoms remain somewhere — dispersed, bonded differently, integrated into other molecules. Biological regeneration gathers atoms from metabolic pools and assembles them gradually.

Matter rearrangement.

But if restoration occurs without observable metabolic sourcing, then either matter is transported rapidly from elsewhere, or matter is reorganized from an undifferentiated state.

He felt the question narrowing toward physics.

Quantum field theory teaches that particles arise from field excitations. The vacuum state is not empty; it contains fluctuating potential. Particle-antiparticle pairs emerge transiently. Fields permeate space.

If fields are fundamental and particles are excitations, then matter is already emergent — not static.

Regeneration at the deepest level would not require external importation of matter.

It would require specification of field excitations.

In other words, matter regeneration would be controlled differentiation of an underlying field.

He wrote it carefully in his notes:

Matter Rearrangement: Repositioning existing atoms or molecules within physical constraints.

Matter Regeneration: Differentiation of underlying field substrate into specified particle configurations.

The second category implied something radical.

If a deeper undifferentiated field exists — a unified substrate from which known fields differentiate — then localized modulation of that substrate could generate specific particle arrangements directly.

This would not violate conservation laws.

Energy would still be required.

But instead of moving atoms from one place to another, structure would emerge from controlled field excitation.

He paused and considered the cosmological parallel.

After the Big Bang, the universe existed in a hot, dense, undifferentiated state. As it cooled, symmetry broke. Particles emerged. Matter condensed. Galaxies formed.

Creation at cosmic scale was not rearrangement.

It was differentiation.

If that process occurred once universally, could it occur locally under specific conditions?

He felt the intellectual tension rising.

Such control would be indistinguishable from creation.

He walked slowly across the underground chamber, watching particle simulations flicker across the curved display.

Matter rearrangement explains wound healing.

Matter regeneration would explain instantaneous structural reinstatement.

He imagined a retinal layer destroyed by injury. Rearrangement would require gradual cell proliferation. Regeneration at field level would require specifying particle states to match the prior structural blueprint.

The visible outcome would appear miraculous.

But the mechanism would be physical.

The distinction between rearrangement and regeneration also clarified the boundary between biological stem cells and his emerging hypothesis.

Biological stem cells rearrange matter gradually.

A Particle Stem Cell — if it exists — would regenerate matter directly.

Not through cell division.

But through field differentiation.

He felt the idea hardening into conceptual architecture.

If biology represents differentiation at cellular scale, and physics represents differentiation at particle scale, then the deepest regenerative capacity must lie beneath both.

An undifferentiated substrate.

He wrote once more in his encrypted journal:

Biological Stem Cell: Undifferentiated cell capable of producing multiple tissues.

Particle Stem Cell: Undifferentiated quantum substrate capable of producing any particle configuration.

The symmetry was too precise to ignore.

The more he examined the architecture of matter, the more it mirrored the architecture of life.

Undifferentiated → Differentiated → Stabilized.

Reversal requires destabilization.

Regeneration requires controlled redifferentiation.

He stopped in front of the display and watched simulated particle interactions shimmer and collapse.

Matter rearrangement is engineering within constraints.

Matter regeneration is engineering of constraints themselves.

The distinction would define everything that followed.

If healing is rearrangement, medicine suffices.

If healing is regeneration at field level, physics must enter the conversation.

And if physics enters the conversation, then the concept of miracles shifts from supernatural to structural.

He leaned back against the console and closed his eyes briefly.

The boundary had been drawn clearly now.

Biology explains rearrangement.

The next chapter would have to confront the possibility of regeneration from undifferentiated substrate.

Which meant he could no longer avoid the central question forming with increasing clarity:

Does an undifferentiated quantum state exist beneath known particle fields?

And if it does...

Is it accessible?

The investigation had reached the edge of conventional science.

Beyond it lay the hypothesis that would define the rest of his work.

The Particle Stem Cell.

And stepping into that hypothesis would require abandoning the safety of biology entirely.

He opened his eyes.

It was time to descend deeper.

Chapter 13

Are Miracles Violations of Nature?

The question had been circling for weeks, though Dr. Myles Darwin had refused to state it plainly.

Now he did.

He stood before his students and wrote across the board:

Are miracles violations of nature — or expressions of deeper law?

The room tightened.

Not because of theology.

Because of structure.

Myles did not approach the question as a believer defending faith or as a skeptic dismantling it. He approached it as a scientist interrogating mechanism.

A violation of nature would imply suspension of physical law. An interruption of causality. An event without mechanism.

But physics, as far as it has advanced, has never encountered a true violation of law. Instead, history reveals a pattern: phenomena once considered supernatural are later explained by deeper understanding.

Lightning was once divine wrath.

It is now electrical discharge.

Disease was once curse.

It is now microbial infection.

The pattern suggests something crucial: when understanding deepens, mystery recedes — not by erasing wonder, but by revealing mechanism.

So if accounts of instantaneous healing exist — whether interpreted literally or symbolically — the correct scientific question is not "Did this violate nature?" but "If this occurred, what law governed it?"

He let that settle.

Because to call something a violation is to stop inquiry.

To call it deeper law is to begin inquiry.

He revisited the categories he had established:

Biological regeneration — gradual, time-bound, cell-based.

Matter rearrangement — atomic repositioning under chemical constraint.

Matter regeneration — differentiation from undifferentiated substrate.

If instantaneous restoration occurred, it would not suspend physics.

It would operate at a layer beneath known biological constraint.

The key insight was this:

Law is layered.

Newtonian mechanics explains macroscopic motion. Quantum mechanics governs particle behavior. Relativity governs spacetime curvature. None violate the others; they operate at different scales.

What appears impossible at one layer may be trivial at another.

For example, quantum tunneling allows particles to cross energy barriers that classical mechanics forbids. At macro scale, tunneling seems impossible. At quantum scale, it is routine.

Scale determines apparent lawfulness.

Myles paced slowly as he spoke.

"If biological law forbids instantaneous tissue reconstruction," he said quietly, "that does not mean physical law forbids it."

It means biological law is not the deepest layer.

He returned to symmetry breaking in early cosmology. The universe began in a high-energy unified state. As energy levels shifted, forces differentiated. Structure emerged. No violation occurred. Only transition.

What appears miraculous at one energy state is normal at another.

He felt the intellectual architecture stabilizing.

Miracles, if literal, would not violate nature.

They would require access to a deeper energy regime or field condition.

And that deeper regime would not contradict known law — it would encompass it.

He wrote in his journal that night:

A miracle is not suspension of law.

It is activation of law at a deeper layer than normally accessible.

The statement disturbed him.

Because if true, it implied accessibility.

If deeper layers of law exist, and if they can be activated intentionally, then humanity could potentially reproduce such events.

Healing would not require divine exception.

It would require understanding.

But understanding at that depth carries consequence.

To manipulate field-level structure is to manipulate matter itself.

He returned again to the distinction between rearrangement and regeneration.

Rearrangement obeys known law.

Regeneration from undifferentiated substrate would require access to a field state beyond currently controlled conditions.

Such a field state might resemble early-universe symmetry — a unified condition from which particles differentiate.

If localized symmetry restoration were possible, then localized redifferentiation would follow.

Structure would shift without violating conservation.

Energy would redistribute.

Matter would reorganize.

He felt both exhilaration and caution rising simultaneously.

If miracles are deeper law, then they are not supernatural.

They are advanced physics.

And advanced physics is replicable.

Replicability erases mystery but amplifies responsibility.

He considered again the hypothetical restoration of sight. If retinal tissue were reinstated through field differentiation, the event would appear instantaneous. But the mechanism would not suspend causality.

It would operate through causality at a deeper scale.

He leaned forward over his desk, fingers interlaced.

There are three possibilities when encountering accounts of instantaneous healing:

1. The account is metaphorical or exaggerated.
2. The event occurred through unknown biological mechanism.
3. The event occurred through activation of deeper physical law.

The first possibility requires no further inquiry.

The second remains within medical advancement.

The third demands physics beyond current reach.

Myles found himself unwilling to dismiss the third possibility purely because it felt uncomfortable.

He did not claim such events occurred.

He claimed only that they would not require suspension of law — only access to deeper law.

And that difference is everything.

He stood once more before the underground particle array and watched simulated field fluctuations ripple across space.

Fields permeate vacuum.

Particles emerge from excitation.

Symmetry breaks and forms differentiate.

What if the undifferentiated state remains accessible — not cosmologically, but locally?

What if the substrate beneath known particle fields is not extinguished by cosmic cooling, but remains as latent possibility?

The idea sharpened into clarity.

If biological stem cells represent undifferentiated potential at cellular scale...

Then a particle stem cell would represent undifferentiated potential at quantum scale.

And if accessed, differentiation could be reinitiated deliberately.

Miracles would not be violations.

They would be technical operations at foundational layer.

He closed his journal slowly.

The question had matured beyond theology.

It had become architectural.

If deeper law governs structure, and if structure can be reinstated by accessing that law...

Then the next logical step is unavoidable:

Does such an undifferentiated quantum state exist?

And if it exists...

Can it be specified?

The semester had now fully crossed into Part III — from miracles reexamined to the architecture of matter itself.

He could no longer linger at the edge.

The Particle Stem Cell Hypothesis awaited articulation.

And once articulated, it would change everything.

Chapter 14

The Architecture of Matter

Dr. Myles Darwin had spent months descending through layers of biological identity. Tissue into cells. Cells into molecules. Molecules into atoms. But now he stood at the edge of something far more fundamental — the architecture of matter itself.

He projected a simple image onto the lecture hall screen: a single hydrogen atom. A proton. An electron. Space between them.

"This," he said quietly, "is not solid."

The room remained still.

The atom, once imagined as the smallest indivisible unit, is mostly emptiness. The nucleus occupies an almost incomprehensibly small fraction of its total volume. The electron does not orbit like a planet but exists as a probability distribution — a wave function describing where it might be observed.

Matter feels solid because of electromagnetic repulsion between electron clouds.

Not because it is dense.

Structure is not substance.

Structure is interaction.

He began peeling the architecture further.

Protons and neutrons inside the nucleus are not fundamental either. They are composed of quarks, bound together by gluons through the strong nuclear force. Quarks themselves are elementary — at least as far as current experiments can measure.

But even these are not "things" in the classical sense.

Modern physics describes reality in terms of quantum fields. Each type of particle corresponds to a field that permeates all of space. The electron field exists everywhere. The quark fields exist everywhere. The photon field exists everywhere.

What we call a particle is simply a localized excitation — a vibration — in its respective field.

The field is fundamental.

The particle is derivative.

Myles let that settle.

Because this was the turning point.

If matter is built from particles, and particles are excitations of fields, then fields are the true substrate of physical reality.

And fields are not localized objects.

They are continuous.

Even in vacuum — even in empty space — these fields exist in a ground state. They fluctuate. They contain latent energy. Virtual particles appear and vanish.

The vacuum is not empty.

It is structured potential.

The pattern echoed too strongly to ignore.

In biology, the stem cell exists in an undifferentiated state, capable of becoming specialized tissue under the influence of regulatory signals.

In physics, the quantum field exists in an undifferentiated ground state, capable of producing particle excitations under the influence of energy and symmetry breaking.

Differentiation at cellular scale.

Differentiation at quantum scale.

He shifted the projection to a diagram of early-universe symmetry. Immediately after the Big Bang, forces were unified. The electromagnetic force and weak force were one. The strong force had not yet separated. As the universe cooled, symmetry broke. Forces differentiated. Particles acquired mass through interaction with the Higgs field.

Mass itself is not intrinsic.

It arises from interaction.

Without the Higgs field, particles would not possess rest mass. They would move at light speed, incapable of forming stable atoms.

Identity, even at the particle level, is relational.

He felt the architecture clarifying in his mind.

Matter is layered:

Fields

→ Particle excitations

→ Atoms

→ Molecules

→ Cells

→ Tissue

→ Organisms

Each layer is a stabilized differentiation of the one beneath it.

At no point does structure arise from nothing.

It arises from underlying potential shaped by interaction.

He walked slowly across the underground facility later that night, particle simulation arrays glowing in curved arcs of light.

If quantum fields are primary and particles are differentiated states of those fields, then the most fundamental layer of matter is not the particle.

It is the field configuration.

And if fields can differentiate under changing conditions...

Could they also be redifferentiated?

The question lingered like gravity.

In cosmology, phase transitions occurred when energy levels dropped below critical thresholds. Fields shifted configuration. Symmetry broke. Structure emerged.

Phase transitions are not gradual.

They are threshold-based.

He leaned closer to the simulation.

If a deeper unified field once existed — a state before current field differentiation — then perhaps beneath known fields lies a more fundamental undifferentiated substrate.

Not electron field.

Not quark field.

But a unified pre-field.

An architectural origin state.

If accessed, that state would not rearrange existing particles.

It would differentiate new particle configurations directly.

Matter would not be shuffled.

It would be specified.

He returned to his earlier hierarchy.

Biological stem cells are not fundamental matter — they are specialized cellular assemblies.

But their behavior reveals a pattern:

Undifferentiated → Instruction → Differentiated structure.

What if matter itself obeys the same architecture?

Undifferentiated quantum substrate → Symmetry breaking → Particle differentiation → Atomic structure.

The architecture of matter was no longer a static pyramid.

It was a dynamic cascade of differentiation.

And differentiation implies reversibility under certain conditions.

He sat down heavily in the chair beneath the simulation display.

If a unified undifferentiated field underlies known quantum fields, then that field would be the "totipotent" layer of matter.

A Particle Stem Cell would not be a particle at all.

It would be the undifferentiated condition of physical reality.

From it, all particle identities could emerge.

He typed slowly into his encrypted journal:

The architecture of matter mirrors the architecture of life.

At its root lies an undifferentiated state.

Differentiation produces identity.

Identity stabilizes structure.

He paused before adding:

If the undifferentiated state can be accessed locally, matter can be regenerated rather than rearranged.

The implications reverberated through him.

This was no longer about healing alone.

If matter is structured differentiation of fields, and if differentiation can be controlled, then creation itself becomes technical.

He powered down the simulation screens one by one.

The architecture was clear now.

Matter is not solid substance.

It is patterned excitation of fields.

And beneath those patterns may lie a deeper undifferentiated architecture — a substrate of potential from which structure differentiates.

The next chapter would demand that he articulate the most dangerous idea yet:

The Undifferentiated Quantum State.

And once named, it could no longer remain theoretical curiosity.

It would become a hypothesis.

The Particle Stem Cell Hypothesis.

The descent was complete.

Now came articulation.

Chapter 15

Quantum Fields and the Birth of Particles

Dr. Myles Darwin had spent years studying cells under microscopes, watching undifferentiated biological potential resolve into muscle, nerve, and blood. But now he stood before something far more unsettling — the realization that matter itself may undergo a similar process.

He projected a single equation onto the wall of the underground facility. It was not dramatic. It was not poetic. It was the mathematical expression of a quantum field.

"Particles," he said softly to the empty room, "are not things."

In classical physics, matter is composed of objects — tiny indivisible units that stack together to form larger structures. But modern quantum field theory dismantled that picture entirely. The fundamental entities of reality are not particles, but fields.

An electron is not a tiny solid sphere orbiting a nucleus.

It is an excitation — a vibration — of the electron field.

A quark is not a microscopic bead.

It is a localized oscillation in the quark field.

Photons are excitations of the electromagnetic field. Gluons arise from the gluon field. Every fundamental particle corresponds to a field that permeates all of space.

The field exists everywhere.

The particle is what happens when the field vibrates.

This was the true architecture of matter.

Fields are continuous. They stretch across the universe. Even in regions devoid of atoms, devoid of stars, devoid of galaxies, the fields remain. The vacuum is not empty. It is a ground state of these fields — a lowest energy configuration that still contains latent activity.

Quantum fluctuations ripple through the vacuum constantly. Virtual particles emerge and annihilate in infinitesimal fractions of time. Potential is not hypothetical.

It is built into the structure of emptiness.

Myles felt the symmetry reappearing once again.

In embryology, the fertilized egg contains the full genomic field of possibility. Differentiation does not introduce new information; it excites specific genes under regulatory signals. Structure emerges from patterned activation.

In physics, the quantum field contains the potential for particle manifestation. Under specific energy conditions, excitations occur. Structure emerges from patterned vibration.

Biology does not invent differentiation.

It reflects it.

He turned the projection toward cosmology.

In the earliest moments after the Big Bang, the universe was in an extraordinarily hot and dense condition. Energy dominated. At such extreme temperatures, distinctions between forces blurred. The electromagnetic and weak forces were unified. The strong force behaved differently. Some theories suggest that at even higher energies, all forces may have been unified in a single field.

As the universe expanded and cooled, symmetry broke.

The unified field differentiated into distinct forces. Particles acquired mass through interaction with the Higgs field. Quarks combined into protons and neutrons. Electrons stabilized. Atoms eventually formed.

The birth of particles was not gradual construction.

It was phase differentiation.

Symmetry breaking is the key.

When a system's energy state changes, the configuration of its fields changes. Under high symmetry, possibilities are broad and undifferentiated. When symmetry breaks, specific stable configurations emerge.

Identity crystallizes from potential.

Myles leaned against the console and watched a simulation of spontaneous symmetry breaking — a visual representation of a field settling into a lower-energy differentiated state. The transformation appeared abrupt. Once a threshold was crossed, the system reorganized rapidly.

The pattern mirrored biology again.

A stem cell remains pluripotent until regulatory thresholds push it toward differentiation. Once a specific gene network stabilizes, identity locks in.

At cosmic scale, the universe remained symmetric until cooling forced differentiation of forces and particles.

The birth of particles was the universe's first act of specialization.

He began mapping the analogy explicitly in his notes:

Biological differentiation:

Undifferentiated cell → regulatory signals → stable specialized identity.

Cosmic differentiation:

Unified field → symmetry breaking → stable particle identity.

The resonance between the two systems was no longer philosophical.

It was structural.

He inhaled slowly.

If particles are differentiated excitations of fields, and if fields themselves differentiated from a unified state, then matter at its root is layered specialization.

Which means specialization is not fundamental.

It is emergent.

He returned to the Higgs field.

Before interaction with the Higgs field, particles would be massless. They would travel at light speed. Stable matter would not form. It is interaction with this pervasive field that gives particles mass — resistance to acceleration.

Mass is not intrinsic.

It is relational.

The deeper Myles descended, the clearer it became: nothing in matter is inherently solid, fixed, or absolute. Everything emerges through interaction with underlying fields.

Particles are not building blocks.

They are stabilized excitations.

And stabilization implies reversibility under altered conditions.

He did not yet claim reversibility was possible.

He only observed that if differentiation occurred once, it is not logically impossible for differentiation to occur again under proper conditions.

The universe differentiated into particles billions of years ago.

What if localized field conditions could induce differentiation again?

What if particle identity is not final, but conditional?

He wrote slowly:

If quantum fields give birth to particles through symmetry breaking, then particle identity is a stabilized outcome of deeper field conditions.

He paused before adding:

A deeper undifferentiated substrate may exist beneath known fields — a pre-differentiated state capable of generating multiple field configurations.

The thought was no longer speculative mysticism.

It was a logical extension of unification physics.

Modern physics continues seeking a Grand Unified Theory — a framework that describes all forces as manifestations of a single underlying interaction. The closer one looks, the more reality appears unified at origin.

Unity precedes multiplicity.

Just as in embryology.

He walked slowly through the dim chamber, particle detection arrays humming softly in the background.

If the birth of particles was the universe's first differentiation event, then the possibility of redifferentiation cannot be dismissed outright.

The blind who saw.

Instant reconstruction.

Matter rearrangement versus matter regeneration.

The Acceleration Hypothesis.

All roads now pointed here.

If matter arises from fields, and fields arise from deeper symmetry, then perhaps beneath the differentiated universe lies an undifferentiated quantum state — not erased by cosmic history, but embedded in its foundation.

And if that state exists...

Then differentiation can, in principle, be invoked.

Not as violation.

But as activation.

He closed his journal for the night.

Quantum fields were no longer abstract mathematics.

They were the womb of matter.

And somewhere within that womb might lie the undifferentiated substrate he had been searching for since he first stared at a stem cell under fluorescence.

The next step would be the most dangerous articulation of all:

To formally propose the Particle Stem Cell Hypothesis.

And once proposed, it would demand evidence.
Because if particles are born from fields...
Then the question is no longer whether differentiation exists.
The question is whether it can be directed.

Chapter 16

Differentiation at the Quantum Scale

Differentiation, Dr. Myles Darwin had come to realize, was not a biological invention.

It was a structural principle of reality.

In embryology, a stem cell differentiates when regulatory signals bias its internal state toward one stable identity among many possibilities. In physics, something eerily similar occurs at scales far beyond biological visibility.

Quantum systems do not begin in fixed states.

They begin in superposition.

An electron, prior to measurement, is not in a single position. It exists as a probability distribution — a wave function describing multiple possible outcomes. Only when interaction occurs does that wave function collapse into a specific measurable state.

Possibility collapses into identity.

Myles stood in the underground facility staring at a simulation of wave function evolution. The probability field shimmered, describing where a particle might exist. When interaction occurred — measurement, collision, entanglement — the distributed potential resolved into a single outcome.

This was not mystical.

It was the mathematics of quantum mechanics.

Before interaction, the system is undifferentiated among its possible states.

After interaction, it is differentiated.

He felt the biological parallel tightening.

A pluripotent stem cell carries multiple potential gene expression programs. Under regulatory influence, it commits to one. The wave function of cellular identity collapses into a stable differentiated state.

At quantum scale, particles emerge from probabilistic fields when interaction stabilizes them into measurable excitations.

Differentiation is the stabilization of possibility.

He began writing slowly in his notebook:

Biological differentiation:

Superposition of gene potential → regulatory interaction → stable cell identity.

Quantum differentiation:

Superposition of probability states → interaction/measurement → stable particle identity.

The structural similarity was unmistakable.

But quantum differentiation extended further.

In early-universe cosmology, differentiation did not merely occur at the level of individual particles. Entire fields underwent symmetry breaking. When temperature dropped below certain thresholds, unified interactions separated into distinct forces.

The electromagnetic force and weak force were once unified as the electroweak force. Only after symmetry breaking did they become distinct interactions.

Before differentiation, there was unity.

After differentiation, specialization.

He turned toward the Higgs field model once more. Particles acquire mass through interaction with the Higgs field. Before that interaction, massless states exist. After interaction, differentiated identity stabilizes.

Mass is not fundamental.

It is a differentiated property.

Myles felt a subtle shift within his thinking.

If differentiation at quantum scale depends on interaction and energy conditions, then particle identity is conditional.

And if conditional, then it is not absolute.

He paced slowly.

Consider phase transitions in condensed matter physics. When temperature drops below critical levels, materials undergo structural reorganization. Superconductivity emerges. Magnetization aligns. Liquid crystallizes into solid.

At threshold, the system differentiates into a new stable configuration.

The process can appear abrupt.

Phase transitions are quantum differentiation at macro scale.

The deeper he examined it, the clearer the pattern became:

- Fields contain undifferentiated potential.
- Energy thresholds trigger differentiation.
- Stable identities emerge.
- Structure persists until conditions change again.

Differentiation is governed by landscape.

Energy landscape.

Probability landscape.

Field landscape.

In biology, gene regulatory networks create landscapes of cellular fate — sometimes visualized as Waddington's epigenetic landscape, where a ball rolls down branching valleys toward stable cell types.

In physics, potential energy landscapes determine which field configurations are stable under given conditions.

The analogy was no longer aesthetic.

It was mathematical.

He wrote:

Differentiation at quantum scale is the collapse of high-symmetry potential into lower-symmetry stable states under changing energy conditions.

Then he paused.

If that is true, then the undifferentiated quantum state must correspond to a high-symmetry configuration — a unified condition in which multiple field possibilities coexist.

In early cosmology, such a state existed.

But does it still exist beneath current differentiated fields?

Modern unification theories — including grand unified models and string-inspired frameworks — suggest that at sufficiently high energies, distinctions between forces dissolve. The universe returns to symmetry.

This implies something crucial:

The undifferentiated condition is not mythological.

It is physical.

It simply requires different energy parameters.

He leaned back and let the implication settle.

If differentiation occurs when symmetry breaks...

Then redifferentiation could occur if symmetry is restored.

He did not mean reversing the entire universe to early Big Bang conditions.

He meant localized symmetry restoration.

Localized reconfiguration of field conditions.

If possible, particle identity could be re-specified.

Matter would not be rearranged atom by atom.

It would be redifferentiated from deeper symmetry.

He felt the weight of the thought deepen.

Biological stem cells differentiate through gene regulation.

Quantum systems differentiate through symmetry breaking and measurement interaction.

If there exists a pre-field undifferentiated quantum state — a foundational substrate — then it would be the totipotent state of matter.

He whispered quietly in the dim chamber:

"Particle identity is not final."

The idea did not violate physics.

It extended it.

Particle identity emerges from field conditions.

Change the conditions, change the identity.

The only obstacle is scale and control.

He returned to the retinal example once more in his mind.

If tissue is composed of atoms, atoms of particles, and particles of field excitations, then differentiation at quantum scale ultimately defines biological structure.

Therefore, biological regeneration is constrained by quantum differentiation.

And if quantum differentiation can be influenced...

Then biological structure can be reinstated from below.

He opened his encrypted journal again.

Differentiation at the quantum scale suggests that particle identity is stabilized but not absolute.

Under specific energy and symmetry conditions, new particle states can emerge.

If controlled, such differentiation could specify matter directly.

He paused before writing the final line for the night:

The Particle Stem Cell would not be a particle.

It would be the high-symmetry undifferentiated quantum state from which particles differentiate.

The semester had now fully crossed into territory that blurred physics and ontology.

Differentiation was no longer confined to cells.

It was woven into the architecture of the universe.

And if differentiation is universal...
Then regeneration is not a biological anomaly.
It is a structural echo of cosmic process.
The next chapter would demand the most radical articulation yet:
To formally define the Particle Stem Cell Hypothesis.
And once defined, it would either collapse under scrutiny...
Or change the way humanity understands matter itself.

Chapter 17

The Undifferentiated Quantum State

Dr. Myles Darwin had descended through biology, through atoms, through quantum fields, and now he stood at the edge of something even more fundamental.

If differentiation occurs at every observable layer of reality, then what lies beneath differentiation itself?

He no longer asked this question rhetorically.

He asked it as a structural necessity.

In early cosmology, there existed a state before particle identity — a high-energy condition in which distinctions between forces had not yet emerged. The universe was symmetric. Unified. Indistinguishable in its interactions. As expansion occurred and energy decreased, symmetry broke. Fields differentiated. Particles acquired identity.

The undifferentiated preceded the differentiated.

But the early universe was not nothing.

It was a state.

A condition of unified field symmetry.

Modern physics suggests that at sufficiently high energies, the known forces of nature — electromagnetic, weak, strong — converge toward unity. Grand Unified Theories attempt to mathematically describe this convergence. At extreme scales, differentiation dissolves.

Unity returns.

This implies something crucial.

The differentiated universe is not the only configuration possible.

It is one phase.

Myles stared at a simulation of symmetry restoration — a theoretical reversal in which increasing energy density forces distinct fields to merge again into unified behavior.

Symmetry breaking created specialization.

Symmetry restoration would dissolve it.

He leaned back slowly.

If such unified conditions existed once, then differentiation is not the absolute baseline of reality.

Unity is.

Differentiation is a stabilized expression of unity under specific energy constraints.

He began outlining the logic carefully in his journal:

1. The universe began in a unified, high-symmetry state.
2. Symmetry breaking produced differentiated fields and particles.
3. Differentiation stabilized into the matter structures we observe.
4. Unified states remain theoretically accessible under sufficient energy conditions.

But the critical question remained:

Is the undifferentiated quantum state merely a historical condition of the early universe?

Or is it structurally embedded beneath current field configurations?

Quantum field theory does not describe fields as created at the Big Bang and frozen afterward. Fields exist everywhere. They permeate spacetime. The vacuum state is not empty; it is the ground configuration of these fields.

The undifferentiated condition may not be absent.

It may be suppressed.

Just as pluripotency in a differentiated cell is suppressed by epigenetic regulation.

That analogy returned with startling clarity.

A skin cell does not lose the genes required to become a neuron. It silences them.

The early universe's unified symmetry may not have vanished. It may have transitioned into a stabilized lower-energy configuration.

The deeper substrate may still exist beneath differentiated fields — inaccessible under ordinary conditions, but structurally present.

He stood and paced slowly.

The undifferentiated quantum state would not be chaos.

It would be maximal symmetry.

Maximal possibility.

In such a state, particle distinctions dissolve. Charges are undefined. Mass is not yet acquired. Interaction types are unified.

It would be the "totipotent" condition of matter.

He felt the weight of the term pressing toward inevitability.

If biological totipotency allows differentiation into any tissue, then quantum totipotency would allow differentiation into any particle configuration.

But accessing such a state is not trivial.

In cosmology, it required energy densities near the origin of the universe. Such energies are not casually produced. They are approached only in high-energy particle accelerators and theoretical early-universe conditions.

However, physics has repeatedly demonstrated that local conditions can emulate cosmological phenomena on small scales. Quantum chromodynamics recreates quark-gluon plasma under extreme collision energies. Particle colliders briefly approach conditions not seen since cosmic infancy.

This means something profound:

The undifferentiated state is not metaphysical.

It is physical.

It simply requires appropriate conditions.

Myles returned to the retina example once more, but now with a refined lens.

If a retinal structure were destroyed, biological regeneration would attempt gradual reconstruction. But if one could locally induce a quantum symmetry restoration — a temporary reaccess to undifferentiated substrate — and then specify redifferentiation into precise particle configurations corresponding to retinal architecture...

The reconstruction would not require time-bound cell division.

It would require controlled differentiation from unified state.

He felt a quiet tremor of realization.

The undifferentiated quantum state is not a particle.

It is not even a field in the conventional sense.

It is the condition before field distinction.

The ground symmetry from which fields differentiate.

He wrote carefully:

The Undifferentiated Quantum State (UQS):

A high-symmetry, unified configuration of quantum substrate in which distinctions between known fields and particle identities are not yet resolved.

He paused.

Then added:

Differentiation from UQS produces known particle types through symmetry breaking.

This was no longer poetic speculation.

It was a conceptual extension of established symmetry principles.

But he recognized the danger immediately.

If the UQS exists and is accessible, then control over differentiation would equate to control over particle identity.

Which equates to control over matter.

He closed his eyes briefly.

Biology taught him that undifferentiated states are powerful but unstable. Pluripotent cells must be tightly regulated to prevent tumor formation.

The undifferentiated quantum state would be infinitely more volatile.

Stability at particle level underpins atomic structure, chemistry, life itself. Disrupt it carelessly, and matter may not reorganize predictably.

And yet, the pattern across scales remained too consistent to ignore.

Life differentiates.

Matter differentiates.

The universe differentiates.

Differentiation implies undifferentiation as origin.

The UQS was not an exotic fantasy.

It was the logical root of symmetry.

He stood in silence beneath the dim hum of superconducting coils and particle detectors.

The blind who saw.

Instant tissue reconstruction.

The Acceleration Hypothesis.

Matter regeneration versus rearrangement.

Quantum differentiation.

All threads converged here.

If miracles are deeper law, then that law resides at the level of undifferentiated quantum symmetry.

He opened his journal once more and wrote the sentence that crystallized everything:

The Particle Stem Cell is the Undifferentiated Quantum State

—

the foundational substrate from which particle identity differentiates.

The hypothesis was now explicit.

Not metaphor.

Not analogy.

A structural claim.

If correct, it would unify biology, physics, and cosmology under one principle:

Undifferentiated potential precedes specialized identity.

The semester had crossed beyond curiosity.

Now it demanded formulation.

The next chapter would formalize the hypothesis completely.

And once formalized, it would no longer be a philosophical exercise.

It would become a challenge to reality itself.

Chapter 18

The Particle Stem Cell Hypothesis

Dr. Myles Darwin did not rush this chapter.

He did not present it to students immediately.

He did not publish it.

He did not even speak it aloud at first.

He wrote it alone.

Because once articulated, it could not be withdrawn.

The logic had unfolded layer by layer:

- Stem cells are undifferentiated biological units capable of generating specialized tissues.
- Differentiation is the stabilization of potential into identity.
- Regeneration is reactivation of latent potential under controlled conditions.
- Matter is not built from rigid particles but from excitations of quantum fields.
- Quantum fields themselves differentiated from a high-symmetry unified state.
- Symmetry breaking is the mechanism of identity formation at cosmic scale.

The pattern repeated too precisely across scales to ignore.

Differentiation is universal.

Therefore, undifferentiation must also be universal.

He began writing carefully:

The Particle Stem Cell Hypothesis proposes that beneath known quantum fields exists a unified undifferentiated quantum

substrate capable of differentiating into any known particle configuration under specific symmetry-breaking conditions.

He stopped.

The sentence felt dangerous.

Because it implied that particle identity is not fundamental.

It is emergent.

If electron, quark, photon, and gluon identities arise through differentiation from deeper substrate, then matter itself is a stabilized expression of deeper potential.

The biological analogy was no longer metaphorical.

It was structural.

In a pluripotent stem cell, multiple genetic pathways coexist in potential form. Regulatory signals push the system into one stable configuration.

In the undifferentiated quantum state, multiple field configurations may coexist in symmetric form. Energy thresholds push the system into one stable differentiated configuration.

He drew a diagram in his notebook:

UQS (Undifferentiated Quantum State)

↓ symmetry breaking

Quantum Fields

↓ excitations

Particles

↓ interactions

Atoms

↓ bonding

Molecules

↓ organization

Cells

↓ differentiation

Tissues

The architecture was continuous.

He exhaled slowly.

If the UQS is the "totipotent" layer of matter, then the Particle Stem Cell is not a new particle species.

It is a condition.

A state of maximal symmetry.

A unified potential from which known particles differentiate.

He refined the hypothesis further:

1. The UQS exists as a high-symmetry configuration beneath known quantum fields.
2. Known particle identities arise through symmetry breaking from this substrate.
3. Under specific energy or field conditions, localized reaccess to UQS may be theoretically possible.
4. Controlled redifferentiation from UQS could specify particle configurations directly.

The fourth statement was the one that changed everything.

If particle configurations can be specified directly, then matter need not be rearranged.

It can be regenerated.

He paused and considered conservation laws.

Energy cannot be created or destroyed.

Momentum must be conserved.

Charge must be conserved.

The hypothesis did not violate these laws.

It required that energy input under specific conditions induces differentiation of unified substrate into stable configurations.

Just as high-energy collisions in particle accelerators produce new particle states.

Creation from field excitation is already known.

The difference would be control.

He leaned back in the chair and closed his eyes.

If this hypothesis is correct, then instantaneous structural reconstruction becomes theoretically plausible.

Not because time is compressed.

Not because biological law is suspended.

But because matter is specified from substrate rather than grown through cells.

The blind who saw would not represent cellular acceleration.

It would represent particle-level redifferentiation.

The lame who walked would not represent muscular regrowth.

It would represent structural reinstatement.

The rabbit from the hat would not be illusion.

It would be field differentiation under controlled conditions.

He opened his eyes again.

The implications extended beyond healing.

If UQS can differentiate into any particle configuration, then:

- Elements can be specified.
- Complex molecular structures can be instantiated.
- Matter can be manifested from unified substrate under energy constraint.

The difference between miracle and engineering collapses.

He felt both awe and dread rising simultaneously.

Because the hypothesis, if true, implies that reality is not fixed.

It is programmable at its root.

But programmability implies vulnerability.

Stabilized matter exists because symmetry remains broken under current energy conditions. Disturb those conditions recklessly, and matter destabilizes unpredictably.

He wrote another line:

The Particle Stem Cell is not a substance to be extracted.

It is a symmetry state to be induced.

That distinction was crucial.

One does not "find" the UQS.

One alters field conditions such that differentiation resets.

He thought again of biological reprogramming. Yamanaka factors do not add new genes. They alter regulatory conditions to unlock suppressed potential.

The Particle Stem Cell Hypothesis suggests a similar mechanism at quantum scale:

Alter field symmetry conditions, and undifferentiated substrate becomes accessible.

Then specify redifferentiation.

He stood and walked slowly to the particle simulation display.

The glowing equations did not argue.

They simply described possibility.

Symmetry breaking is real.

Field unification is real.

Particle differentiation is real.

The only leap was control.

He spoke softly to the silent chamber:

"If symmetry can break... symmetry can restore."

And if symmetry can restore, differentiation can restart.

He returned to his journal and finalized the chapter's core statement:

The Particle Stem Cell Hypothesis asserts that the undifferentiated quantum substrate remains structurally embedded beneath known fields and that under specific engineered conditions, localized access to this substrate would allow direct differentiation into specified particle configurations, enabling matter regeneration rather than rearrangement.

He underlined one word.

Engineered. Because this was no longer theology.

It was physics extended.

The semester had now crossed into explicit territory.

There was no turning back.

The hypothesis existed. The next step would be to examine its consequences.

Because if matter can be regenerated from undifferentiated substrate...

Then magic is not illusion. It is undeveloped science.

And the age of manifestation would not begin with mystics.

It would begin with engineers.

Chapter 19

Geometry as the Language of Creation

Dr. Myles Darwin did not begin this chapter with equations.

He began with shapes.

A circle.

A triangle.

A square.

A cross.

Projected against the wall of the underground facility, they appeared almost childish in their simplicity. No quantum equations. No field tensors. No symmetry groups. Just pure geometric form.

Yet geometry precedes biology.

Geometry precedes chemistry.

Geometry precedes atoms.

Because before matter becomes substance, it becomes arrangement.

And arrangement is geometry.

He stood silently before the shapes and allowed the realization to deepen.

Every particle interaction can be described geometrically. Field configurations are geometric distributions in spacetime. Symmetry breaking is geometric instability. Atomic orbitals are geometric probability densities. Crystal lattices are geometric repetition. Molecular bonds form geometric angles.

Even DNA is geometry — a double helix defined by spatial configuration.

Creation is not merely energetic.

It is geometric.

He walked slowly to the projection and drew a point at the center of the circle.

A point has no dimension.

Yet it defines position.

From a point, a line can extend. From a line, a plane. From a plane, volume.

Dimensionality unfolds from geometric relationships.

He felt the connection tightening.

If matter is field excitation, and fields are spatial distributions, then geometry is the visible signature of field behavior.

Particles are geometric events in field space.

Biological cells are geometric organizations of molecular fields.

The universe itself expands geometrically.

Geometry is not decoration.

It is structure.

He wrote in his journal:

Energy differentiates through geometry.

The triangle, square, and circle were not symbolic ornaments. They represented fundamental symmetries.

The circle — continuous symmetry.

The triangle — minimal structural stability.

The square — orthogonal order.

The cross — intersection of axes.

Each form represents constraints.

Constraints produce structure.

Without geometric constraint, energy disperses uniformly. No form stabilizes.

Geometry restricts possibility into shape.

He returned to the Undifferentiated Quantum State in his mind.

In maximal symmetry, geometry is uniform. No preferred direction. No distinction.

When symmetry breaks, geometry differentiates. Axes emerge. Orientation appears. Structure stabilizes.

Creation, then, is geometric differentiation of energy.

The more he examined it, the clearer the sequence became:

Undifferentiated energy

→ Geometric symmetry

→ Symmetry breaking

→ Structured geometry

→ Particle stabilization

→ Atomic arrangement

→ Molecular architecture

→ Cellular form

Geometry bridges physics and biology.

He thought of Platonic solids — tetrahedron, cube, octahedron, dodecahedron, icosahedron. Ancient philosophers believed these shapes represented elemental structure. Though modern chemistry superseded literal interpretations, the intuition was not misplaced.

Matter organizes in geometric patterns.

Even quantum mechanics is described using geometric mathematics — Hilbert spaces, symmetry groups, manifolds.

The language of creation is not narrative.

It is geometry.

He approached the central display and overlaid a simulation of field oscillation with geometric grid lines. The patterns aligned with remarkable clarity. Nodes formed at intersection points. Oscillations followed geometric constraints.

Field differentiation produces geometric stability.

And geometric stability produces identity.

He paused and recalled his earlier drawing — the convergence of elementary shapes into a unified geometric symbol.

If simple geometric primitives can combine into more complex forms, then geometry itself behaves like differentiation.

The point is undifferentiated position.

Lines differentiate direction.

Planes differentiate dimension.

Volumes differentiate structure.

Geometry evolves through constrained expansion.

He wrote carefully:

If the Undifferentiated Quantum State is maximal symmetry, then geometry emerges as the first differentiation.

This was crucial.

Before particle identity, before mass, before charge — spatial differentiation must occur.

Spacetime curvature itself is geometric.

General relativity describes gravity not as force, but as geometry of spacetime.

Creation is geometric deformation of underlying substrate.

He exhaled slowly.

If geometry is the language of creation, then specifying geometry is specifying structure.

Which means the Particle Stem Cell Hypothesis requires geometric instruction.

One does not merely induce undifferentiated state.

One specifies the geometry into which it differentiates.

The retina is not merely atoms.

It is layered geometry.

Muscle tissue is not merely molecules.

It is aligned geometric pattern.

If matter is programmable, the code must be geometric.

He felt the conceptual architecture locking into place.

Biology supplies blueprint.

Physics supplies substrate.

Geometry supplies specification.

He wrote one final line for the chapter:

Energy differentiates through geometry. Geometry stabilizes identity. Identity becomes matter.

The shapes still glowed faintly on the wall.

Circle.

Triangle.

Square.

Cross.

They no longer appeared simple.

They appeared foundational.

The next chapter would examine something even more personal — his own geometric convergence system.

Because if geometry is the language of creation, then perhaps a unified geometric stem symbol could reflect the undifferentiated substrate itself.

And if symbols mirror structure...

Then mathematics may be closer to matter than previously imagined.

The descent into geometry had begun.

And geometry never lies.

Chapter 20

Convergence of Elementary Forms

Dr. Myles Darwin did not approach geometry as an artist; he approached it as a physicist who had reached the limits of language. Equations described behavior, fields described interaction, and symmetry described transformation, but geometry described structure, and structure is what survives differentiation. He stood before the projection of the simple shapes once more — circle, triangle, square, cross — and slowly began layering them. At first, they remained separate, distinct, independent forms. Each carried its own symmetry group and represented a different structural constraint. The circle represented rotational symmetry with no preferred axis. The triangle represented minimal stability, the simplest polygon capable of enclosing space. The square represented orthogonality, right angles and stability within grid systems. The cross represented intersection, the meeting of axes and the birth of coordinate systems. Individually, they were elementary. Together, they began to do something unexpected: they converged.

As he overlaid the shapes onto a single central point, something remarkable occurred. The boundaries blurred, the symmetries interacted, lines intersected, axes multiplied, and rotational symmetry collided with angular stability. Complexity emerged from convergence — not addition, but convergence. He paused, recognizing that convergence is not accumulation; it is alignment. When elementary forms align at a shared origin, they cease to be separate and become unified geometry. He zoomed in on the central point where all forms intersected. That point — dimensionless and structureless — anchored all geometry. Without it, no line could extend, no plane could rotate, no symmetry could exist. The point was the undifferentiated geometric state from which all forms differentiated.

He felt the resonance immediately. The Undifferentiated Quantum State was analogous to the geometric point. It contains no dimension, no orientation, no distinction, yet from it all structured geometry emerges. He wrote carefully in his journal that the geometric point is the undifferentiated origin of form, and that convergence of elementary shapes at a point reflects differentiation from unified state. The deeper he examined the convergence, the clearer the structural truth became. When a triangle is inscribed within a circle, constraints interact; when a square is rotated within that circle, additional axes appear; when cross-lines extend through the center, coordinate orientation emerges. From convergence, higher-order symmetry arises, and symmetry is what stabilizes identity. In particle physics, symmetry groups define allowable interactions, gauge symmetries determine force behavior, and the mathematics of particle physics is fundamentally geometric. Group theory — the study of symmetry transformations — underpins the Standard Model. Reality is written in symmetry operations.

He paced slowly, considering that if elementary geometric forms represent fundamental symmetries, then their convergence at a shared origin reflects the possibility of unified symmetry. The circle alone represents infinite rotational symmetry; the triangle introduces discrete symmetry; the square introduces orthogonal axes; the cross introduces directional polarity. When converged, they no longer compete — they integrate. The result is not chaos but structured complexity. He began to see something more profound: if geometry converges at a single origin point, then differentiation is simply divergence from that point. All forms are variations of constraint applied to origin. All letters, numbers, symbols — even language itself — can be decomposed into geometric primitives.

He paused and considered his own constructed system — the unified geometric stem symbol that contained within it the potential to generate all letters and numbers through rotational and structural manipulation. It was not artistic invention; it was structural recognition. Convergence at origin allows infinite differentiation, just as the Undifferentiated Quantum State allows infinite particle differentiation. He felt the intellectual bridge solidifying: biology shows that a stem cell contains potential for all tissue types, physics shows that the undifferentiated quantum state contains potential for all particle types, and geometry shows that a central point contains potential for all forms. Convergence is the act of holding all elementary constraints in unified equilibrium, and from that equilibrium differentiation produces variety.

He leaned forward and whispered, "The origin contains the universe." Not metaphorically, but geometrically. The point contains all directions. The undifferentiated state contains all symmetries. The stem cell contains all tissue potential. Convergence is not compression; it is unity before divergence. He wrote slowly in his journal that convergence of elementary forms mirrors unification of quantum fields, differentiation of forms mirrors symmetry breaking, and the geometric stem symbol is a structural analogue of the Particle Stem Cell. He stopped writing and stared at the symbol again. It was not mystical; it was inevitable. When elementary forms align at a shared origin, complexity becomes generative rather than chaotic. The more he examined it, the clearer it became that geometry is not merely descriptive — it is generative. Mathematics does not describe reality passively; it defines allowable structures. Particle interactions obey group symmetries because geometry governs possibility.

He felt the implications expanding. If geometry is the language of creation, then convergence is the grammar. The undifferentiated state is the root, differentiation is syntax, and matter is sentence. He allowed himself a rare moment of stillness, recognizing that convergence of elementary forms is not decorative abstraction but structural necessity. The universe did not begin with scattered shapes; it began with unified symmetry. Differentiation produced diversity. He turned off the projection slowly, and the shapes faded into darkness, but the point remained in his mind — invisible, dimensionless, infinite in potential. The next chapter would push this convergence further, because if geometric convergence mirrors quantum unification, then perhaps mathematics itself is not an invention but a discovery of structural truth embedded in matter. And if so, the geometric stem symbol is not merely representation — it may be reflection. The descent into geometry had become irreversible, and the origin was no longer abstract. It was foundational.

Chapter 21

The Omni Decimal System

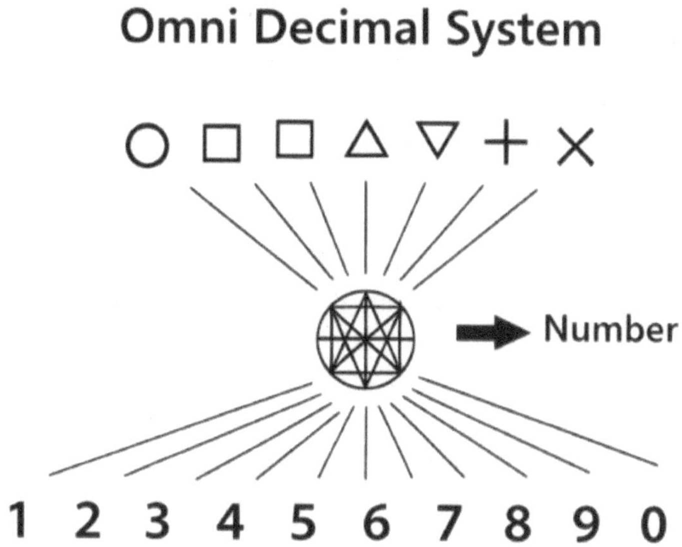

DR. MYLES DARWIN NO longer saw numbers as symbols created for counting; he saw them as compressed geometry. After confronting convergence at the level of elementary forms, he began asking a more radical question: if geometry is the language of creation, then what is arithmetic? What is number? Numbers had always appeared abstract, detached from matter, yet every measurable property of the universe is expressed numerically. Charge is quantified. Spin is quantized. Energy levels are discrete. The constants of nature are numerical ratios. The universe does not merely contain numbers — it behaves numerically.

He stood before the projection screen once more, but this time instead of shapes, he displayed the digits zero through nine. At first glance they appeared culturally arbitrary, historical artifacts of human notation. Yet when he stripped them down to their geometric essence, each digit could be decomposed into curves, angles, intersections, and closed loops. A zero is a circle. A one is a vertical axis. A two curves into angular redirection. A three repeats curvature. A four anchors orthogonality. A five bends symmetry. A six and nine mirror rotational inversion. An eight is stacked infinity compressed into dual circles. Every digit is geometry constrained into recognizable form.

The decimal system itself — base ten — is not random. It is positional. Each place value represents multiplication by powers of ten. Structure arises not from the digit alone but from its position relative to origin. A one placed left or right of a decimal transforms magnitude exponentially. Value is geometric placement in abstract space. Number is positional symmetry.

He began sketching his unified geometric stem symbol beside the digits. If elementary geometric forms converge at a single origin, and if all letters and numbers can be derived through rotational manipulation of that unified form, then number is not separate from geometry — it is differentiated geometry. The Omni Decimal System, as he began calling it privately, was not merely a counting mechanism. It was a reflection of convergence expressed numerically.

In traditional mathematics, zero represents absence. Yet geometrically, zero is not emptiness — it is enclosure. It is the circle. It is containment without differentiation. It is potential before magnitude. Without zero, positional notation collapses. Without the circle, no closed system stabilizes. Zero is not nothing; it is origin framed.

One represents direction. Two introduces polarity. Three introduces stability. Four establishes dimensionality. Five breaks symmetry. Six curves expansion. Seven tilts balance. Eight loops infinity into finite enclosure. Nine approaches completion before returning to zero in cyclical renewal. Ten is not merely one plus zero; it is unity returning to origin at higher order.

He felt something profound unfolding. The decimal cycle is geometric recurrence. After nine, the sequence does not invent new shapes; it repositions existing ones. Ten reintroduces one at a higher magnitude. One hundred repeats one within expanded positional geometry. The decimal system is convergence scaled through place value.

He wrote slowly in his journal that the Omni Decimal System is not simply numerical convenience but structural recursion. Each digit is a geometric variation emerging from a unified stem configuration, and positional notation is differentiation through spatial displacement. Just as particle differentiation emerges from symmetry breaking, numerical magnitude emerges from positional shift.

He began examining the deeper pattern. Mathematics describes physical law because mathematics reflects geometry, and geometry reflects field structure. When physicists write equations describing quantum states, they are not inventing reality — they are mapping geometric relationships. Group symmetries define particle behavior. Constants emerge as stable ratios within geometric constraint. Number is not external to matter. It is embedded in its architecture.

If geometry is the grammar of creation, then number is its syntax. The Omni Decimal System represents cyclical convergence returning to origin while expanding magnitude. Each numerical cycle mirrors differentiation from unity and return to unity at higher order. Zero to nine is a full geometric sweep; ten resets at expanded scale. The system is recursive unity.

He paused before the projection and considered something unsettling. If numbers are geometric differentiations of unified origin, and if the unified geometric stem symbol contains the generative pattern for all numeric forms, then arithmetic itself may be a shadow of deeper symmetry. The universe calculates because it is structured. It measures because it is geometric.

Biology counts cell divisions. Physics quantizes energy. Chemistry balances equations. Everywhere he looked, number governed structure. And if the decimal system reflects geometric recurrence, then the Omni Decimal System becomes more than symbolic design. It becomes structural mirror.

He leaned back and whispered softly that convergence of elementary forms generates geometry, geometry generates number, and number governs matter. The chain was no longer philosophical; it was architectural. If the Undifferentiated Quantum State is the origin of particle identity, and if geometry is the first differentiation of that state, then number may be the quantized expression of geometry itself.

He stared at the digits once more — zero through nine — and no longer saw arbitrary symbols. He saw constrained curves and angles emerging from unified structure. He saw recursion. He saw symmetry. He saw return. The Omni Decimal System was not invented; it was discovered within structural possibility.

And if number is embedded in geometry, and geometry in field symmetry, then mathematics is not human creation alone. It is recognition.

The next step would push the idea further still, because if geometry generates number and number describes matter, then perhaps language itself — letters, symbols, codes — are differentiated expressions of the same unified stem. And if that is true, then convergence does not stop at shape or digit.

It extends into meaning.

The descent was no longer about physics alone. It was about structure itself.

Chapter 22

The Stem Symbol

By the time Dr. Myles Darwin turned his full attention to the stem symbol, it no longer felt like invention. It felt like inevitability. After tracing differentiation from biology to quantum fields, from symmetry to geometry, from geometry to number, he began to see that convergence demanded representation. Not decorative representation, not mystical abstraction, but structural condensation. If the Undifferentiated Quantum State was the foundational substrate of matter, and if geometry was its first visible differentiation, then there must exist a geometric configuration capable of symbolizing unified potential before divergence. That configuration became the stem symbol.

He stood before the projection screen in the underground facility and displayed the converged elementary forms once more: circle, triangle, square, and cross layered upon a single central origin. Yet now he refined the structure further. He aligned the axes with precision, balanced rotational symmetry against angular stability, ensured orthogonality intersected curvature without distortion. The result was not chaotic overlap. It was equilibrium. Every constraint held tension against another. Every line referenced the center. The origin was preserved as the anchor of all differentiation.

The stem symbol was not merely the sum of its parts. It was the equilibrium state from which all parts could be derived. Rotate the configuration and one form becomes emphasized. Shift orientation and another emerges. Remove certain constraints and letters begin to appear. Adjust proportion and numerical shapes reveal themselves. It was generative without being unstable. It was unified without erasing distinction. It was convergence embodied.

He traced its central point slowly with his finger across the projection. That point contained no dimension, yet it structured every dimension around it. From that origin extended axes, from axes emerged planes, from planes arose enclosures, and from enclosures stabilized recognizable form. The symbol behaved exactly like the geometric analogue of the Undifferentiated Quantum State. Before specialization, there is unity. After divergence, identity appears. The stem symbol held unity without collapsing into abstraction.

He began writing carefully in his journal that the stem symbol is the geometric analogue of quantum totipotency. It contains within a single unified configuration the structural potential for multiple differentiated forms. Just as a biological stem cell contains genetic pathways for multiple tissue identities, and just as the undifferentiated quantum substrate contains potential for multiple particle configurations, the stem symbol contains geometric pathways for letters, numbers, and structural expressions. It is not a symbol in the artistic sense; it is a convergence map.

The more he examined it, the more the pattern revealed itself. Language reduces to geometry. Letters are combinations of curves, angles, and intersections. Numbers are rotational manipulations of arcs and lines. Codes are sequences of constrained forms. All symbolic systems ultimately reduce to spatial differentiation. The stem symbol was not meant to replace alphabets or numeric systems; it revealed their shared origin. It demonstrated that divergence from unity produces recognizable complexity without losing structural coherence.

He felt something profound in that recognition. Symbols across civilizations have attempted to capture unity before multiplicity — circles representing eternity, intersecting lines representing balance, geometric mandalas expressing symmetry. But the stem symbol was not mystical iconography. It was structural synthesis. It emerged from studying symmetry groups, field differentiation, and geometric constraint. It was architecture, not ornament.

Standing alone in the dim chamber, Myles realized the symbol also carried something more subtle. It was stable. Remove any one element, and the equilibrium shifted. Overemphasize one axis, and symmetry broke prematurely. True convergence required balance. The stem symbol demonstrated that unity is not homogeneity; it is equilibrium of constraints. This mirrored physics precisely. The early universe's unified symmetry was not chaos. It was balanced interaction before differentiation.

He whispered quietly that the stem symbol is not representation of matter but reflection of its logic. The Undifferentiated Quantum State represents maximal symmetry; symmetry breaking produces differentiation; differentiation stabilizes into identity. The symbol compresses that sequence into geometric form. It is the grammar of convergence held at rest.

He began imagining further implications. If geometry is generative and the stem symbol encodes convergence, then specifying geometric differentiation could become a method of structural instruction. Not mystical invocation, but mathematical precision. If particle identity emerges through symmetry breaking, and if geometry defines symmetry, then the stem symbol may represent the equilibrium condition prior to differentiation. It would not create matter, but it would mirror the pattern through which matter becomes.

He closed his journal slowly and allowed the projection to fade into darkness. The symbol remained in his mind, hovering as a silent convergence of possibility. It was no longer merely a drawing. It was a bridge between abstraction and substrate, between mathematics and matter, between unity and multiplicity.

The next step would be unavoidable. If the stem symbol reflects convergence at geometric level, and if convergence mirrors quantum unification, then the question becomes more than symbolic. It becomes operational. Can convergence be induced beyond representation? Can geometry move from reflection to instruction?

The descent had reached a new depth. The symbol was no longer decorative. It was foundational. And somewhere within its equilibrium lay the possibility that structure itself could be spoken into differentiation — not by magic, but by symmetry understood.

Chapter 23

Alphabetic Differentiation

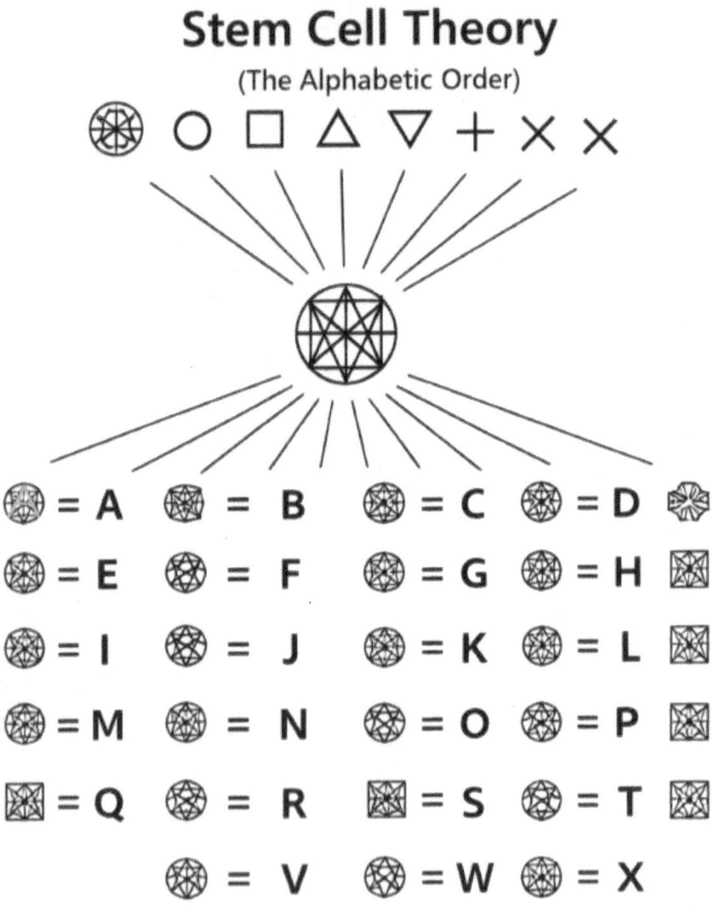

BY THE TIME DR. MYLES Darwin turned toward language itself, he no longer saw letters as arbitrary markings invented by culture. He saw them as differentiated geometry. After tracing convergence from quantum symmetry to geometric form and from geometric form to numerical structure, the next logical descent was into alphabet. If numbers were quantized expressions of geometric recurrence, then letters were directional expressions of geometric differentiation. Language, he began to suspect, was not separate from structure — it was structured divergence from a unified origin.

He projected the alphabet onto the wall of the underground facility and began stripping the letters down to their skeletal forms. The curves of "C" and "S" reduced to arcs of a circle. The straight lines of "E" and "F" reduced to orthogonal axes. The diagonals of "A" and "V" revealed angular stability. The enclosure of "O" returned to circular unity. The intersection of "T" and "X" revealed polarity and crossing symmetry. There was no letter that could not be decomposed into lines, curves, and intersections — the same elementary geometric constraints he had already studied. The alphabet was not invention; it was rotation and restriction of geometric primitives.

He felt the structural resonance deepen. The stem symbol, with its converged circle, triangle, square, and cross anchored at a central origin, already contained the potential for all directional variation. Rotate the symbol and a vertical line emerges. Emphasize curvature and an arc appears. Extend one axis and suppress another and angular differentiation forms. Letters were not created independently; they were geometric selections from unified possibility.

Alphabetic differentiation, he realized, mirrors quantum differentiation. Just as a unified quantum substrate differentiates into specific particle identities under symmetry breaking, a unified geometric stem differentiates into letters under constraint selection. The origin remains constant. The differentiation changes orientation, proportion, and emphasis. Identity emerges from geometric bias.

He began writing slowly in his journal that alphabetic forms are constrained rotations and extensions of unified geometry. Each letter represents a stabilized configuration of lines and curves selected from converged symmetry. The alphabet is not random; it is differentiated structure. When a child learns to write, they are not inventing lines — they are reproducing geometric decisions that emerged from centuries of structural refinement.

He paced slowly, contemplating the deeper implication. Language is not merely sound mapped to symbol. It is geometry mapped to meaning. The shapes of letters are stabilized forms capable of encoding thought because they are structured. Structure allows repeatability. Repeatability allows communication. Communication allows civilization. Geometry sits beneath meaning like a silent foundation.

The comparison grew sharper. In biology, differentiation produces tissues that carry specialized functions — muscle contracts, neurons transmit, epithelial layers protect. In language, differentiation produces letters that carry specialized phonetic functions — vowels open, consonants constrain, combinations generate words. The stem symbol, holding all geometric potential at equilibrium, mirrors the undifferentiated state before linguistic specialization.

He considered something even more profound. Across cultures, alphabets differ in appearance but not in principle. Whether Latin, Greek, Hebrew, Arabic, or Cyrillic, all scripts reduce to combinations of lines and curves. Even logographic systems such as Chinese reduce to constrained strokes arranged within spatial rules. The geometry changes style, but the principle of differentiation from primitive forms remains constant. Unity gives rise to multiplicity through constraint.

Alphabetic differentiation therefore becomes more than artistic design. It becomes structural echo of the same process that governs particle identity. Just as symmetry breaking determines allowable particle states, geometric constraint determines allowable letter states.

The alphabet is a field of possible forms stabilized by tradition and repetition.

He leaned closer to the projection and whispered softly that language itself is a differentiated field. Letters are excitations within that field. Words are composite particles formed by structured combinations. Sentences are molecules of thought. Meaning emerges through relational geometry of symbols in sequence. Just as atoms combine under chemical laws, letters combine under grammatical laws.

He felt the intellectual bridge solidifying further. Biology differentiates from stem cell. Physics differentiates from unified field. Geometry differentiates from origin point. Number differentiates from positional structure. Alphabet differentiates from geometric primitives. The pattern was recursive across scale.

The stem symbol now appeared even more significant. It was not simply a geometric convergence; it was a generative seed. From it, letters could be derived through rotation, emphasis, and constraint. It behaved like an alphabetic totipotent state. The undifferentiated geometric configuration held within it the structural capacity for linguistic expression.

He wrote in his journal that alphabetic differentiation mirrors symmetry breaking in quantum fields. Unified geometry, when constrained directionally, produces stabilized symbolic identity. The process is not mystical. It is architectural. The same rules that stabilize particle identity stabilize written form.

He stepped back from the projection and allowed the alphabet to fade from the wall. In its place, the stem symbol reappeared silently in his mind. He understood now that language was not separate from matter. Both arise from structured differentiation. Both depend on geometry. Both stabilize identity through constraint.

The implications were expanding beyond physics. If geometry underlies particle identity and also underlies symbolic language, then perhaps meaning itself is not disconnected from structure. Perhaps thought, matter, and language share a common architectural origin in symmetry and differentiation.

The next chapter would force him to confront an even more daring question. If alphabetic forms differentiate from unified geometry, and if geometry mirrors quantum symmetry, then could instruction — spoken or written — one day intersect with matter at structural level? Could language, in some distant future of engineering precision, become not merely descriptive but directive?

The descent into structure had reached language itself. And language, he now understood, is geometry speaking.

Chapter 24

One Symbol, Infinite Expressions

By the time Dr. Myles Darwin arrived at the conclusion forming quietly beneath his research, it no longer felt speculative. It felt structural. After tracing differentiation from quantum symmetry to geometry, from geometry to number, and from number to alphabetic form, the pattern had become undeniable. Unity precedes multiplicity. Convergence precedes divergence. Structure precedes expression. And if that is true across every scale examined, then a single unified configuration must contain within it the potential for infinite expressions.

He returned to the stem symbol once more — the converged geometry of circle, triangle, square, and cross unified at a central origin. He no longer saw it as layered shapes. He saw it as equilibrium. Each constraint balanced another. Rotational symmetry coexisted with angular stability. Orthogonality intersected curvature without conflict. Directional axes emerged without collapsing circular unity. The symbol did not favor one form; it held them all in tension.

It was not complexity through accumulation. It was complexity through balance.

He began manipulating the symbol slowly. Rotate it ninety degrees, and certain axes become dominant. Emphasize curvature and suppress angular extension, and arcs take precedence. Extend one vector while diminishing another, and recognizable letters begin to appear. Shift proportion slightly, and numerical forms emerge. The transformations were not forced. They were latent. The symbol did not resist differentiation; it permitted it.

He leaned back and realized something profound: infinite variation does not require infinite starting forms. It requires one sufficiently unified origin.

Just as the Undifferentiated Quantum State contains the potential for all particle identities through symmetry breaking, the stem symbol contains the potential for all geometric expressions through constraint modulation. One symbol does not limit diversity; it enables it. Multiplicity is not contradiction of unity. It is its expression.

He wrote carefully in his journal that a unified geometric equilibrium can produce infinite expressions through directional bias, proportional shift, rotational orientation, and constraint emphasis. The stem symbol is not a static image but a generative seed. It does not depict a letter, a number, or a particle; it contains the structural capacity to become any of them.

The deeper he considered it, the clearer the recursive pattern became. In biology, one fertilized cell differentiates into trillions of specialized cells. In physics, one unified symmetry differentiates into distinct forces and particles. In mathematics, one set of axioms generates infinite theorems. In language, a finite alphabet generates infinite sentences. Infinity does not require infinite origin; it requires generative structure.

The stem symbol was generative structure embodied.

He stared at the central point of the symbol again. The origin did not change when differentiation occurred. The point remained constant while forms radiated outward in variation. That constancy was the key. Identity emerges from divergence, but origin remains untouched. Just as quantum fields differentiate while underlying spacetime persists, just as stem cells specialize while genetic code remains embedded, just as numbers cycle while zero anchors the system, the symbol's center held equilibrium while expression unfolded.

He whispered quietly that one symbol can contain infinite expressions because unity is not absence of diversity; it is the ground of it.

The more he examined the transformations, the more he realized that differentiation does not destroy the original symbol. It reveals pathways within it. Each new form is not an addition from outside; it is a selection from within. Infinite expressions are not imported. They are unlocked.

He began to sense the deeper implication for the Particle Stem Cell Hypothesis. If the Undifferentiated Quantum State is unified equilibrium of symmetry, then differentiation into particles is not external creation. It is structural expression. Matter is not built from foreign addition; it unfolds from unified substrate.

The stem symbol was not a metaphor anymore. It was a mirror.

He paced slowly through the dim chamber, the glow of simulation arrays reflecting off the walls. If one unified geometric configuration can produce infinite symbolic forms, then perhaps one unified quantum substrate can produce infinite material forms. The scale changes. The principle does not.

He wrote again that infinite expression from single origin is not mystical — it is architectural inevitability wherever symmetry, constraint, and generative rules coexist.

The implication widened beyond geometry. It touched language, physics, biology, mathematics, and perhaps even consciousness itself. Unity does not eliminate difference. It enables it. Infinite variation is stabilized divergence from equilibrium.

He stood still for a moment, understanding that the stem symbol was not the final answer but the structural demonstration of a deeper truth. One symbol, infinite expressions. One field, infinite particles. One stem cell, infinite tissues. One origin, infinite universe.

The next question could no longer be avoided. If unity contains infinite expression, then differentiation must be governed by rule. And rule implies law. If the stem symbol reflects lawful differentiation of form, then the Undifferentiated Quantum State must obey lawful differentiation of matter.

The descent had reached the threshold where philosophy meets engineering. Because if one unified structure can produce infinite expression, then the future will not be about discovering new building blocks. It will be about understanding the generative rules embedded in the original one.

And once those rules are understood, expression will no longer be accidental. It will be intentional.

Chapter 25

The Rabbit and the Hat

Dr. Myles Darwin did not begin this chapter in a laboratory or beneath particle simulations. He began it in a theater. A stage. A spotlight. A magician holding an empty hat before an audience certain of impossibility. The rabbit appears. Applause erupts. The illusion is complete. Yet what fascinated Myles was not the trick itself, but the structural question beneath it: why does the human mind instinctively label sudden manifestation as magic?

The rabbit was not in the hat, the audience believes. Therefore, its appearance violates expectation. But expectation is merely a model of process. We assume that objects require continuity of movement, gradual transition from one location to another, visible cause preceding visible effect. When that continuity is hidden or bypassed, we call the result supernatural.

He sat quietly in his office later that evening and rewrote the scene in structural terms. There are only three possible explanations for the rabbit's appearance. First, it was physically hidden within the hat or stage mechanism. Second, it was transported from another location through concealed means. Third, it was instantiated at the location. The first two rely on rearrangement. The third implies regeneration.

The human mind rejects the third because it contradicts everyday experience. Matter does not normally appear without visible sourcing. Yet at quantum scale, particles constantly emerge from field fluctuations. Virtual particle pairs appear and annihilate within vacuum states. High-energy collisions produce matter from energy according to conservation laws. The birth of particles is not fantasy; it is measured fact.

The difference between stage illusion and particle physics is not possibility. It is scale and control.

If the Undifferentiated Quantum State exists as unified substrate beneath differentiated fields, and if symmetry breaking differentiates particle identities, then instantiation of matter is not metaphysical. It is field differentiation under energy constraint. The rabbit in the hat becomes a metaphor for particle-level regeneration rather than biological rearrangement.

He leaned back and considered the deeper parallel. In traditional magic, the illusion depends on concealed mechanism. The magician never violates physics; he manipulates perception. In advanced physics, concealed mechanisms also operate — vacuum fluctuations, symmetry breaking, quantum tunneling — phenomena invisible to ordinary senses yet entirely lawful.

What if future engineering bridged the gap between theatrical illusion and quantum law? What if localized field manipulation allowed controlled differentiation of unified substrate into complex structures? The rabbit would not be hidden. It would be specified.

He wrote slowly in his journal that the rabbit and the hat symbolize the human misunderstanding of manifestation. We assume continuity because we experience only macroscopic causality. But deeper layers of reality operate through threshold transitions. Phase changes occur abruptly. Symmetry breaking produces rapid stabilization. Differentiation can appear instantaneous when viewed from higher scale.

The rabbit does not violate nature; it violates expectation.

He walked to the particle simulation array and watched virtual excitations flicker in and out of existence. The vacuum was not empty. It was potential suppressed beneath stability. If energy input destabilizes symmetry locally, differentiation occurs. Matter emerges. The universe has performed this act since its beginning.

The difference between illusion and engineering lies in intentionality. The magician conceals mechanism to create wonder. The engineer reveals mechanism to create reliability. If the Particle Stem Cell Hypothesis is correct, then matter instantiation would not rely on concealment but on precision. The hat would not hide the rabbit; the field would specify it.

He felt a subtle shift in the philosophical weight of the idea. Ancient accounts of sudden materialization — whether mythic, religious, or folkloric — might not represent suspension of law but activation of deeper law beyond everyday access. The human mind calls what it cannot explain "magic." Science calls it "mechanism awaiting discovery."

He whispered softly that the rabbit and the hat are not opposites of physics. They are incomplete models of it.

If geometry is the language of creation, and if symmetry governs differentiation, then instantiation is lawful transformation of undifferentiated substrate into structured matter. The hat becomes localized boundary conditions. The rabbit becomes specified configuration. The illusion becomes threshold event.

He paused, recognizing the danger embedded in such reasoning. The difference between demonstration and catastrophe at quantum scale is precision. Controlled symmetry breaking produces stable particles. Uncontrolled symmetry destabilization destroys structure. Manifestation is not trivial. It is regulated by conservation and energy thresholds.

Still, the structural parallel remained. Matter is not fundamentally solid. It is stabilized excitation. Stabilized excitation can, in principle, be induced.

He closed his journal and let the thought settle. The rabbit in the hat is not a childish trick. It is a symbolic doorway into deeper architectural possibility. What appears from nothing may simply emerge from unified potential under altered symmetry.

The next chapter would move beyond metaphor. If manifestation is lawful differentiation, then the question becomes technological. How would one engineer the field conditions necessary to induce controlled redifferentiation?

Because once the rabbit is no longer illusion but specification, the stage is no longer theater. It is laboratory.

And the hat is no longer cloth. It is symmetry waiting to break.

Chapter 26

Matter Transfer Theory

Dr. Myles Darwin understood that instantiation was only one possible explanation for the rabbit in the hat. If matter could be differentiated from undifferentiated substrate, then manifestation was theoretically plausible. But there was another possibility that required no regeneration at all — only relocation. The rabbit may not have been created. It may have been transferred.

He sat before the simulation arrays and began examining the concept of transfer not at biological scale, but at quantum scale. In classical physics, matter transfer requires motion through space. An object moves from one coordinate to another along a continuous path. Velocity, acceleration, and time govern its trajectory. But quantum mechanics had already fractured this intuition. Quantum tunneling allows particles to appear on the other side of energy barriers without traversing the space between in classical terms. Entanglement connects particles across distance in ways that defy local realism. At fundamental scale, spatial continuity is not always required in the way macroscopic intuition demands.

He leaned forward and whispered that relocation does not necessarily mean traversal.

Matter Transfer Theory began forming in his mind as an alternative branch of the Particle Stem Cell Hypothesis. Instead of inducing undifferentiated substrate to regenerate matter locally, one might alter field conditions such that a structured configuration in one location becomes destabilized and re-stabilized elsewhere. Not creation. Not annihilation. Reconfiguration across boundary conditions.

The key was understanding matter not as solid blocks but as field excitations. If particles are excitations of quantum fields, and if those fields permeate all of spacetime, then spatial separation may not be as absolute as classical physics implies. A particle at one location is not isolated from the field; it is a localized excitation within a continuous substrate.

He began sketching the idea slowly in his journal. Suppose a structured configuration — say, a biological organism — is composed of trillions of stabilized excitations across multiple fields. If one could map the field configuration precisely, one could theoretically suppress that configuration in one spatial region while inducing an identical configuration in another region of the same underlying field. The total field energy remains conserved. The excitation pattern shifts locality.

The organism would not travel through intervening space. The excitation pattern would reappear at a new coordinate.

To an observer, it would resemble teleportation.

He paused, aware of the staggering complexity of such a mechanism. The precision required would exceed any current technological capacity. The informational mapping alone would be astronomical. But structurally, the theory did not violate physics. Field excitations already emerge and collapse under varying energy conditions. Pair production already converts energy into particle structure. Quantum states already demonstrate nonlocal correlations.

The difference between theory and feasibility lay in control.

He paced slowly through the chamber, recognizing that Matter Transfer Theory required two foundational capabilities. First, the ability to encode and preserve the geometric and field configuration of complex matter with extreme precision. Second, the ability to induce controlled symmetry shifts in distant regions of the field substrate to recreate that configuration faithfully.

It was not enough to copy geometry. One must copy phase relationships, quantum states, energy distributions, and boundary conditions. Any deviation could destabilize structure catastrophically.

He exhaled slowly and considered the deeper philosophical implication. Matter transfer does not create something from nothing. It conserves structure by relocating excitation patterns. The rabbit in the hat may not be instantiated from undifferentiated quantum state; it may be re-specified from a distant region of the same field continuum. The hat becomes boundary condition; the stage becomes coordinate transformation.

The idea mirrored certain theoretical constructs in advanced physics. Holographic principles suggest that information about a volume of space can be encoded on its boundary. Quantum information theory treats particles as information-bearing excitations. If matter is fundamentally information encoded in field geometry, then transfer becomes re-encoding rather than movement.

He wrote carefully that Matter Transfer Theory proposes relocation of structured field excitations through coordinated suppression and induction across spatially continuous quantum substrate. Conservation laws remain intact. Energy balances. Charge balances. Structure is not violated; it is recontextualized.

He leaned back and felt the weight of the concept. Instantiation and transfer were not mutually exclusive. They were branches of deeper symmetry manipulation. One differentiates from unified substrate; the other relocates differentiated structure through field continuity. Both rely on understanding matter as excitation, not object.

He stared at the simulations flickering across the walls and whispered that space itself may be less barrier and more topology. If fields permeate all coordinates, then locality is relative stability, not absolute isolation. Matter remains where field conditions stabilize it. Alter the conditions, and stability shifts.

The implications extended beyond spectacle. Medical transport without movement. Resource relocation without shipping. Even environmental restoration through structured rebalancing of field excitations. Yet the same mechanism could destabilize planetary matter if misapplied.

He closed his journal slowly. The rabbit in the hat no longer seemed trivial. It represented two pathways: regeneration from undifferentiated substrate or transfer through field reconfiguration. Both required mastery of symmetry. Both required geometric precision. Both required energy discipline.

The next chapter would force him to confront the most daunting question yet. Whether through instantiation or transfer, control over matter at field level implies technological interface. How does one speak to the substrate? How does one encode geometric instruction into quantum fields?

Because theory alone does not manifest rabbits.

Interface does.

Chapter 28

Miniature Portals and the Retrieval Hypothesis

Dr. Myles Darwin understood that manifestation could be approached in more than one way. Instantiation from undifferentiated substrate was one pathway. Matter transfer through field reconfiguration was another. But there remained a third structural possibility that refused to disappear from his mind — retrieval through localized spacetime manipulation. If matter could not be created without cost and if relocation through field encoding required extreme informational precision, perhaps the simplest explanation for sudden appearance was neither creation nor transfer of excitation pattern, but connection.

He sat before the curved display and called up models of spacetime curvature from general relativity. Gravity, according to Einstein, is not a force in the traditional sense but the curvature of spacetime geometry caused by mass-energy. Massive objects distort the fabric of spacetime, altering trajectories of matter and light. Geometry governs motion. But if spacetime can curve, the question becomes unavoidable: can it fold?

Theoretical physics had long entertained the concept of wormholes — solutions to Einstein's field equations that allow distant regions of spacetime to connect through a shortened geometric pathway. These are not fantasy constructs; they emerge mathematically as permissible configurations under extreme conditions. The problem has never been theoretical allowance. It has been stability. Wormholes, if they exist, would require exotic energy densities to remain open. Without stabilization, they collapse instantly.

Myles leaned forward and whispered that connection does not require traversal through ordinary distance. It requires geometric adjacency.

The Retrieval Hypothesis began forming in his journal as a localized, controlled version of spacetime folding. Instead of regenerating matter from undifferentiated quantum substrate or relocating excitation patterns through field manipulation, one could theoretically create a microscopic bridge between two coordinates. The rabbit does not appear from nothing. It is fetched from elsewhere. The hat is not container. It is gateway.

He wrote slowly that miniature portals would not be large, cinematic tunnels through space. They would be transient geometric distortions in the underlying fabric of spacetime, stabilized for fractions of a second. During that interval, boundary conditions between two locations merge. Matter passes not by traveling through distance but by occupying shared topology.

From the outside, it would resemble sudden appearance. From the inside, it would be retrieval.

He felt the weight of the energy requirements immediately. Spacetime manipulation at meaningful scale demands extraordinary densities. Black holes demonstrate that curvature can become extreme, but they do so under catastrophic gravitational collapse. Controlled curvature without destruction would require energy regulation far beyond present engineering. Yet theoretical permissibility remained. General relativity does not forbid localized curvature manipulation; it merely imposes constraints.

He paced slowly through the dim chamber, recognizing the pattern again. Geometry governs differentiation. Geometry governs number. Geometry governs matter. Geometry governs spacetime itself. If symmetry breaking differentiates particles and if field excitation stabilizes structure, then curvature modifies adjacency. The rabbit may not need to be generated or transferred through field encoding. It may simply be adjacent for an instant.

He imagined a microscopic portal opening between a rural field and a stage. The rabbit, unaware of geometric realignment, steps forward. The boundary closes. Applause follows. No creation. No annihilation. Only temporary adjacency.

He wrote carefully that the Retrieval Hypothesis proposes transient localized spacetime curvature enabling direct adjacency between distant coordinates, allowing matter relocation without conventional traversal. Conservation laws remain intact. Energy input balances curvature. Matter remains continuous with its origin.

The implications widened quickly. Retrieval does not alter particle identity. It does not require undifferentiated quantum state. It requires geometric manipulation at spacetime level. In a sense, it may be simpler than instantiation, though no less energy-intensive.

He paused and considered quantum entanglement again. While entanglement does not allow information transfer faster than light, it demonstrates that spatial separation does not eliminate relational connectivity at fundamental scale. The universe may not be as disconnected as macroscopic intuition suggests. If relational geometry underlies spacetime, then adjacency is conditional.

He whispered softly that space is not distance; it is structure.

Miniature portals would not violate nature. They would exploit geometric permissibility within Einstein's equations. Just as particle accelerators exploit quantum field equations to produce exotic states, advanced curvature engineering would exploit spacetime geometry.

He recognized the danger immediately. Instability in curvature could produce catastrophic gravitational gradients. Energy miscalculation could collapse the portal inward. Retrieval requires stabilization of topology at microscopic scale with precision beyond anything humanity has yet achieved.

Still, the structural possibility remained elegant. Of the three hypotheses — instantiation from undifferentiated substrate, matter transfer through field reconfiguration, and retrieval through miniature portals — none required suspension of physical law. Each required mastery of deeper layers of it.

He closed his journal slowly and stared at the projection of warped spacetime grids glowing faintly in the dark. The rabbit and the hat were no longer stage trick. They were boundary problem. If adjacency can be manipulated, then appearance is geometric event.

The next question loomed heavier than before. Whether through regeneration, transfer, or retrieval, each pathway required interface — a means of speaking to geometry, symmetry, and field. Without interface, the hypotheses remain theory. With interface, they become engineering.

And engineering always asks the same thing: who controls the curvature, who specifies the differentiation, who stabilizes the bridge?

Because once portals are no longer metaphor, distance is no longer protection.

Chapter 29

The Elemental Stem Cell

By the time Dr. Myles Darwin arrived at what he began calling the Elemental Stem Cell, the convergence of all previous chapters felt inevitable. Biology had introduced the stem cell as undifferentiated potential within living systems. Physics had revealed quantum fields as substrates of particle identity. Geometry had exposed convergence as the structural principle underlying differentiation. Manifestation had branched into instantiation, transfer, and retrieval. Yet beneath all of these remained a deeper layer — not merely the Undifferentiated Quantum State in abstract symmetry, but the practical bridge between symmetry and matter itself. That bridge was elemental structure.

He sat in the underground facility studying the periodic table projected across the wall. Hydrogen, helium, carbon, oxygen, iron — each element defined by proton number, electron configuration, quantum behavior. Chemistry rests upon these distinctions. Biology rests upon chemistry. Civilization rests upon elemental manipulation. Yet the periodic table, for all its diversity, is built from only a handful of fundamental particles arranged in specific geometric and energetic configurations.

The realization struck him with clarity: elements are not fundamental. They are stabilized differentiations of particle arrangements.

If that is true, then elemental identity is conditional.

The Elemental Stem Cell hypothesis did not propose a new biological entity. It proposed a structural condition at the level of elemental formation — a controllable state between undifferentiated quantum substrate and stabilized atomic configuration. Where the Particle Stem Cell referred to unified quantum symmetry, the Elemental Stem Cell referred to controlled differentiation into atomic architecture.

He leaned forward and whispered that atoms are frozen symmetry decisions.

An element exists because a specific number of protons stabilize within a nucleus under strong nuclear force, balanced by electron configurations under electromagnetic interaction. Change the proton count and the element changes. Alter the configuration and chemical properties transform entirely. Yet all elements are composed of the same foundational excitations — quarks, electrons, gluons — differentiated through arrangement and quantity.

The Elemental Stem Cell would therefore represent a transitional state in which particle differentiation is stabilized enough to form atomic nuclei, but flexible enough to allow controlled specification of elemental identity before full stabilization. It would not be pure undifferentiated quantum symmetry, nor fully locked atomic structure. It would be an intermediary zone of programmable atomic formation.

He wrote carefully in his journal that the Elemental Stem Cell is a controllable transitional configuration between unified quantum substrate and fixed atomic identity, allowing directed stabilization into chosen elemental forms under precise symmetry and energy conditions.

The idea was radical yet structurally consistent. In nuclear physics, particle accelerators already transmute elements through high-energy collisions. Artificial isotopes are produced. Nuclear reactions alter atomic identity. Stars themselves function as elemental factories, fusing hydrogen into helium and heavier elements through gravitational confinement and extreme temperatures. Elemental change is not fantasy. It is cosmic routine.

The difference between stellar fusion and Elemental Stem Cell engineering would be precision and locality. Instead of brute-force collision or gravitational collapse, one would induce controlled symmetry differentiation at the threshold where proton number stabilizes. One would not smash atoms apart; one would guide their formation.

He paced slowly through the dim chamber, recognizing the implications expanding rapidly. If elemental identity can be specified, then resource scarcity transforms. Metals could be formed without mining. Rare isotopes could be generated without decay chains. Environmental restoration could occur by restructuring elemental contamination at foundational level.

Yet the danger matched the promise. Uncontrolled elemental differentiation could destabilize nuclear binding energies. Miscalculated transitions could release catastrophic radiation. The strong nuclear force does not tolerate approximation. Precision becomes survival.

He returned again to the stem symbol in his mind. Convergence of geometry produces structured differentiation. Similarly, convergence of particle excitations under symmetry constraint produces elemental stabilization. The Elemental Stem Cell is not biological, not purely quantum, but atomic. It is the seed state of matter before periodic table crystallizes into fixed identity.

He whispered quietly that hydrogen was once only symmetry, and iron was once only potential. Stars perform elemental differentiation without consciousness. Engineering would require understanding the same rules with discipline.

He wrote again that the Elemental Stem Cell bridges quantum symmetry and chemical identity. It is the programmable threshold at which proton number, electron configuration, and nuclear stability are specified rather than inherited from natural processes.

The pattern repeated once more across scale. Biology has stem cells that differentiate into tissue. Physics has unified fields that differentiate into particles. Chemistry has elemental formation that differentiates into atomic identity. At each layer, there exists a transitional state where identity is not yet fixed. That transitional state is the stem principle at that scale.

He leaned back slowly, feeling the magnitude of the structure he was building. The Particle Stem Cell addresses matter at its most fundamental. The Elemental Stem Cell addresses matter at its chemical foundation. Together, they describe two tiers of programmable reality — one beneath particles, one at atomic formation.

The next step would extend this principle outward again. If elements can be specified, then complex molecular structures become accessible. If molecules become accessible, then biological regeneration moves from theory to method.

The descent was complete. The ascent toward application was beginning.

And at the center of it all remained the same pattern: unity, differentiation, stabilization.

The Elemental Stem Cell was no longer speculation.

It was the threshold where physics becomes matter by decision.

Chapter 30

Alchemy Reinterpreted

Dr. Myles Darwin never dismissed alchemy as mere superstition. He understood that history often encodes intuition long before science provides mechanism. Ancient alchemists sought the transmutation of base metals into gold, the philosopher's stone, the elixir of life. Modern chemistry rejected their mystical language but quietly achieved what they could not articulate: elemental transformation, isotope manipulation, nuclear synthesis. The dream was not foolish. The framework was incomplete.

Standing before the periodic table glowing softly across the wall, Myles began to reinterpret alchemy not as primitive chemistry but as misunderstood physics. The alchemists believed that matter possessed hidden unity — that beneath apparent differences between lead and gold there existed a deeper sameness that could be unlocked. They were correct in principle. Lead and gold differ only by proton number. Alter the nuclear configuration and one becomes the other. The difficulty was not philosophical; it was energetic.

He wrote slowly in his journal that alchemy sought elemental differentiation without understanding the forces governing nuclear stability. The alchemist searched for a catalyst, a stone, a symbolic convergence that would unlock transformation. Modern physics discovered the catalyst was not mystical powder but nuclear energy. The philosopher's stone was not mineral but symmetry manipulation.

The Elemental Stem Cell hypothesis reframed alchemy entirely. Instead of smashing atoms through brute-force collision as particle accelerators do, the aim would be controlled stabilization at the threshold of elemental formation. The alchemist's furnace becomes a field chamber. The crucible becomes geometric boundary condition. Fire becomes energy input calibrated with precision.

He paced slowly, considering the language of the ancients. They spoke of purification, refinement, dissolution, coagulation. These were metaphors for phase transitions. Dissolution mirrors symmetry destabilization. Coagulation mirrors symmetry breaking into stable identity. Refinement mirrors removal of unstable configurations. Purification mirrors equilibrium restoration. The symbolism was poetic description of structural processes not yet understood.

He leaned forward and whispered that alchemy was geometry without mathematics.

The old texts spoke of one substance underlying all matter — prima materia. Modern physics speaks of unified fields and undifferentiated quantum states. The vocabulary differs, but the intuition converges. Beneath differentiated forms lies unified potential.

The transmutation of metals, once mystical ambition, is now a technical fact. Particle accelerators can convert mercury into gold under specific conditions. Nuclear reactors transmute elements through neutron capture. Stars forge heavier elements from lighter ones in thermonuclear cores. Alchemy did not fail because transformation was impossible; it failed because it lacked precision and energy control.

The reinterpretation, therefore, was not romantic revival. It was structural correction.

He wrote that alchemy reinterpreted through the Elemental Stem Cell framework becomes controlled elemental differentiation guided by geometric and energetic precision rather than symbolic ritual. The philosopher's stone becomes mastery of symmetry thresholds. The elixir of life becomes regenerative stabilization at atomic and molecular scale.

He paused, recognizing the weight of that sentence. If elemental identity can be specified and if molecular architecture can be stabilized directly from geometric instruction, then biological aging itself may be reconsidered. Cellular decay is accumulation of molecular instability. Correct the instability at elemental threshold and structure restores.

Yet he was careful not to drift into fantasy. Nuclear forces are unforgiving. Binding energies are not negotiable. Any attempt at controlled elemental differentiation demands extraordinary accuracy. The strong force does not tolerate approximation. Miscalculation releases radiation, not gold.

He stood in silence for a moment and considered the deeper symmetry once more. Biology contains stem cells capable of tissue renewal. Physics contains unified fields capable of particle differentiation. Chemistry contains elemental thresholds capable of atomic specification. At each level, there exists a transitional state between undifferentiated potential and stabilized identity. Alchemy sought to manipulate that transitional state without understanding its constraints.

He whispered softly that the dream was right; the tools were wrong.

Modern science does not mock alchemy; it fulfills it under stricter discipline. Where alchemy used metaphor, physics uses equation. Where alchemy used furnace, physics uses accelerator. Where alchemy sought gold, physics seeks symmetry.

He closed his journal slowly. The reinterpretation did not romanticize the past. It clarified it. The alchemist's instinct toward unity beneath multiplicity aligns with the Particle Stem Cell hypothesis. The difference is that modern understanding places transformation within conservation law and geometric constraint.

The next question loomed quietly in his mind. If alchemy can be reinterpreted as controlled elemental differentiation, then the boundary between matter and life becomes thinner still. Because once elemental identity can be specified, molecular architecture becomes programmable.

And once molecular architecture becomes programmable, biology is no longer grown.

It is written.

The descent into ancient ambition had revealed not superstition, but premature insight.

And now, armed with geometry and field theory, humanity stands closer to the crucible than ever before.

Chapter 31

3D Printing: Mechanical Precursor

Dr. Myles Darwin did not look to particle accelerators first when imagining the future of matter specification. He looked to something far more ordinary — a 3D printer quietly building a plastic object layer by layer on a desktop. The machine was not mystical. It did not bend spacetime or access undifferentiated quantum states. It extruded filament according to digital instruction. Yet within its mechanical simplicity lay a profound principle: matter can be shaped directly from code.

He stood watching the printer head glide along precise coordinates, depositing heated polymer in microscopic increments. An object that did not exist minutes earlier emerged from structured layering. There was no artisan sculpting it by hand. There was no gradual assembly of separate parts. There was instruction, geometry, and material deposition. The object was not discovered; it was specified.

He whispered softly that 3D printing is geometry made mechanical.

The printer does not invent shape. It reads a digital model — a geometric file composed of coordinates, vectors, and surfaces. The code defines boundaries. The machine obeys. Matter follows instruction within constraints of material properties. The result is a solid form produced directly from information.

He felt the connection tighten immediately. If the Particle Stem Cell Hypothesis proposes that matter at its deepest level is differentiable through symmetry and field conditions, then 3D printing represents a macroscopic analogue of that principle. It is a crude but visible precursor. Instead of accessing unified quantum substrate, the printer manipulates pre-existing material. Instead of symmetry breaking at particle scale, it deposits polymer at positional coordinates. But the architectural logic is identical: geometry directs matter.

He wrote slowly in his journal that 3D printing is a mechanical precursor to field-level matter specification. It demonstrates that structured information can produce physical form without traditional assembly. The machine does not "build" in the classical sense; it manifests structure by following geometric instruction.

He leaned back and considered the deeper implication. A 3D printer requires three essential components: material substrate, energy input, and encoded geometry. Remove any one and the object cannot form. The same triad echoes throughout his research. The Undifferentiated Quantum State provides substrate. Energy induces differentiation. Geometry specifies structure.

In mechanical printing, plastic filament serves as substrate. In advanced engineering, undifferentiated field symmetry would serve as substrate. The printer head deposits material according to code; symmetry breaking would differentiate particles according to geometric constraint. The analogy was no longer poetic — it was procedural.

He paced slowly through the chamber, imagining future iterations. Current printers deposit plastic. More advanced systems deposit metals, ceramics, biological tissue scaffolds. Bioprinters already construct organ-like structures by layering living cells in controlled patterns. The transition from mechanical fabrication to biological regeneration has already begun. The trajectory is clear.

He whispered that the only difference between mechanical printing and elemental differentiation is scale and substrate.

The mechanical printer rearranges matter that already exists. It cannot alter atomic identity. It cannot generate new elements. It cannot rewrite field symmetry. But it proves the principle that geometry governs manifestation. Once digital instruction becomes precise enough and substrate becomes sufficiently flexible, the boundary between fabrication and regeneration blurs.

He imagined a future device not limited to extruding filament but capable of manipulating elemental thresholds directly. Instead of depositing plastic, it would induce localized symmetry conditions that stabilize atomic configurations as specified by geometric code. Instead of building layer by layer from external material, it would differentiate structure from controlled elemental stem states.

He wrote carefully that 3D printing is the mechanical ancestor of elemental differentiation. It is proof that matter can be shaped by information. The future leap is not conceptual; it is technological.

He stood before the glowing screens and considered how natural processes already perform forms of biological "printing." Embryonic development layers tissues according to genetic code. Protein synthesis assembles amino acids according to RNA templates. DNA replication duplicates molecular geometry with astonishing precision. Nature has always been a printer. It simply operates at molecular scale.

The distinction between natural and artificial printing collapses under structural examination. Both require code. Both require substrate. Both require energy. The difference lies in mastery.

He felt the implications widening beyond manufacturing. If biological organs can be printed mechanically, and if elemental identity can be specified through controlled symmetry, then organ regeneration may one day bypass both donor scarcity and slow cellular proliferation. Instead of growing a heart over months, one could specify its geometry and induce structural stabilization at atomic threshold.

He paused, aware of the ethical weight rising with the technological vision. Mechanical printing is harmless when limited to tools and prototypes. Field-level printing would alter the foundation of matter itself. The greater the control, the greater the responsibility.

He whispered quietly that 3D printing is not about plastic. It is about proof of principle. Geometry directs matter. Information becomes form. Code becomes structure.

He turned off the printer and watched the completed object cool into stability. It had not existed before. Now it did. It was not miraculous. It was instructed.

The next step in the descent toward reality's substrate would examine something even more intimate. If mechanical printing is precursor, and elemental differentiation is threshold, then biological regeneration through printing becomes bridge between physics and life.

The future will not begin with particle accelerators.

It will begin with printers.

And eventually, the printer will no longer require filament.

It will require symmetry.

Chapter 32

Bioprinting Organs

Dr. Myles Darwin did not need to imagine the future entirely from theory; parts of it were already unfolding in laboratories across the world. Bioprinting had begun as an experimental extension of mechanical 3D printing, replacing plastic filament with living cells suspended in bio-ink. Layer by layer, researchers were constructing rudimentary tissues — cartilage, skin grafts, vascular scaffolds. The process was still fragile, imperfect, limited in scale. Yet the principle was undeniable: living structure could be printed.

He stood before a projection of a bioprinter depositing thin layers of cellular material into a lattice framework. The machine moved with quiet precision, guided by a digital model derived from medical imaging data. Each droplet of bio-ink contained viable cells arranged according to geometric instruction. After printing, the structure matured in a controlled environment, allowing cells to integrate and stabilize.

He whispered softly that biology has already accepted geometry as command.

In traditional transplantation, organs are harvested from donors. In regenerative medicine, stem cells are coaxed into differentiating over time. Bioprinting merges these approaches. Instead of waiting for natural growth to shape tissue, geometry guides placement immediately. The printer becomes architect; the cells become responsive material.

He wrote slowly in his journal that bioprinting demonstrates the convergence of code, geometry, and living substrate. Digital instruction determines spatial arrangement. Living cells respond to their positional context. Structure emerges from controlled layering.

He paused, reflecting on how closely this mirrored his broader hypothesis. In the biological stem cell, differentiation occurs through signaling gradients and environmental cues. In bioprinting, those gradients are engineered through spatial design. The printer does not change genetic code; it changes geometry. Geometry alters behavior. Behavior stabilizes identity.

He paced slowly, recognizing that bioprinting sits at a critical midpoint between mechanical fabrication and elemental differentiation. It does not manipulate quantum fields or atomic thresholds. It rearranges pre-existing cells. Yet it proves something essential: complex biological systems can be reconstructed through spatial specification rather than organic growth alone.

He leaned forward and studied a model of a printed kidney scaffold. The vascular network — intricate, branching, fractal — was the primary challenge. Without proper blood flow integration, tissue dies. Life depends not only on structure but on dynamic exchange. Printing an organ is not merely about shape; it is about function embedded within geometry.

He whispered that life is geometry in motion.

The more he studied it, the clearer the transition became. Bioprinting currently relies on biological stem cells as substrate. The next step would be printing biological stem cells from elemental thresholds. The future progression seemed almost sequential: mechanical printing rearranges inert matter, bioprinting rearranges living cells, elemental differentiation specifies atomic identity, and Particle Stem Cell engineering accesses undifferentiated substrate.

Each step descends deeper toward structural origin.

He wrote carefully that bioprinting organs is proof that biological complexity can be reconstructed through geometric instruction. It validates the stem principle at macroscopic scale. It shows that regeneration need not rely solely on natural proliferation; it can be directed spatially.

Yet he was acutely aware of limitations. Bioprinting cannot yet replicate full organ complexity with complete vascular integration and neural connectivity. Cells behave unpredictably under stress. Immune rejection remains risk. Time is still required for maturation. The process is guided, but not instantaneous.

He leaned back and considered the contrast between biological and elemental regeneration. Bioprinting is constructive. It layers cells gradually. Elemental differentiation would be immediate stabilization of atomic configuration. The difference is temporal. One grows; the other manifests.

He whispered softly that bioprinting is rehearsal for something deeper.

If geometry can guide living cells into functional organs, then geometry may one day guide atomic differentiation into fully structured biological systems without gradual growth. The heart printed layer by layer today may tomorrow be specified at elemental threshold and stabilized instantly.

He closed his journal and stared at the glowing vascular network rotating slowly on the screen. Bioprinting represents hope within current technological boundaries. It saves lives. It restores function. It proves that structure can be commanded.

But it also reveals the direction of travel. From mechanical precursor to biological architecture to elemental specification, the path is descending toward unified substrate.

The next chapter would force him to confront the ethical and philosophical gravity of that descent. If organs can be printed, and if elements can be specified, and if undifferentiated quantum symmetry can be accessed, then life itself becomes programmable.

And programmability changes everything.

Chapter 33

From Particle to Organ

Dr. Myles Darwin stood alone beneath the dim light of the underground facility and traced the full arc of his inquiry for the first time without interruption. What began as a question about stem cells had descended through tissue, molecule, atom, particle, field, symmetry, and geometry. Now the direction of thought reversed. If the descent had been logical, then the ascent must be equally coherent. If matter differentiates from unified substrate, and if geometry governs stabilization, then the path from particle to organ is not mystical — it is structural.

He began visualizing the chain slowly. Particle excitations stabilize into atomic nuclei through strong nuclear interaction. Atoms bind into molecules through electromagnetic configuration. Molecules assemble into macromolecules through chemical bonding and spatial compatibility. Macromolecules organize into organelles within cells. Cells differentiate into tissues. Tissues integrate into organs. Organs coordinate into organisms. The complexity increases, but the principle does not change. At each level, structure emerges through constrained interaction.

He whispered quietly that life is stabilized geometry layered across scale.

The organ is not separate from the particle. It is particle arrangement extended through hierarchy. A human heart is not mystical flesh. It is atomic configuration shaped by genetic instruction, biochemical constraint, and geometric order. Strip it down far enough and it is quarks arranged into protons, protons into nuclei, nuclei into atoms, atoms into molecules, molecules into cells, cells into muscle fibers aligned with astonishing symmetry.

If particle identity can be specified through controlled symmetry breaking, and if elemental identity can be stabilized through elemental stem states, then molecular architecture becomes programmable. If molecular architecture becomes programmable, cellular identity becomes accessible. If cellular identity becomes accessible, tissue formation becomes directed. And if tissue formation becomes directed, organ construction follows naturally.

He wrote carefully in his journal that the transition from particle to organ is continuous differentiation governed by symmetry, geometry, and energy constraints. There is no discontinuity in principle between quantum excitation and biological complexity; only scaling of structured interactions.

He paced slowly, aware of the magnitude of what he was articulating. Modern medicine treats organs as biological wholes. Bioprinting arranges cells spatially. Genetic engineering modifies molecular code. Yet each of these operates above the elemental threshold. The Particle Stem Cell Hypothesis suggests intervention beneath them — at the level where matter identity is specified.

From particle to organ becomes not evolutionary accident but directed architecture.

He leaned forward and considered the retina once more — the original question that ignited his inquiry. A retina is layered photoreceptors, bipolar cells, ganglion cells, vascular support, neural connections. Each component is molecular geometry stabilized by atomic identity. If atomic identity can be specified and molecular geometry directed, then retinal structure becomes reconstructible without waiting for cellular proliferation.

He whispered softly that regeneration is upward causation from deeper specification.

In nature, the upward chain is slow because each layer waits for the one beneath to stabilize. Atomic bonds form gradually. Molecules self-assemble through probabilistic interactions. Cells differentiate through gene expression over time. Growth obeys chemical kinetics. But if lower layers can be specified intentionally rather than probabilistically, the time dimension compresses dramatically.

He paused, careful not to overreach. Compression does not mean violation. It means direct specification instead of sequential emergence.

He imagined a future chamber not filled with polymer filament or bio-ink but with controlled energy fields calibrated to induce elemental differentiation into predefined molecular lattices. Proteins would not self-assemble through random collision; they would stabilize directly under geometric instruction. Cellular membranes would not grow; they would emerge from specified lipid arrangements. Muscle fibers would align according to directed field constraints.

The organ would not be grown from seed. It would be specified from foundation.

He felt both awe and caution rising in equal measure. The complexity of living systems is not merely structural; it is dynamic. An organ is not only shape but function — electrical signaling, metabolic exchange, adaptive response. Specifying structure is necessary but insufficient without specifying interaction.

He wrote slowly that from particle to organ requires not only atomic arrangement but preservation of functional gradients — electrical, chemical, mechanical. The heart must beat. The lung must exchange gases. The brain must propagate signals. Geometry is necessary but life demands dynamic stability.

He stepped back and allowed the full ladder of differentiation to settle in his mind once more. Unified quantum symmetry differentiates into particles. Particles stabilize into atoms. Atoms bond into molecules. Molecules assemble into living systems. At no point does the principle change. Differentiation under constraint produces identity.

He whispered quietly that life is symmetry extended through time.

The ascent from particle to organ was no longer speculative imagination. It was structural inevitability if control at foundational levels became precise enough. The only barriers were energy discipline, geometric accuracy, and ethical restraint.

He closed his journal and stared into the quiet hum of the facility. The journey had begun with a question about healing. It now touched the architecture of life itself.

The next chapter would confront the inevitable tension that follows such possibility. If organs can be specified from particle foundation, if matter can be directed from unified substrate, then control becomes the defining variable.

And control demands governance.

Because the power to move from particle to organ is not merely medical.

It is civilizational.

Chapter 34

Generating Biological Stem Cells from Elementary Substrate

Dr. Myles Darwin understood that the transition from particle to organ could not leap directly from atomic specification to full biological complexity without an intermediate anchor. Nature itself does not move from quark to heart in a single motion. It stabilizes a transitional state — the biological stem cell. The stem cell is not yet muscle, not yet nerve, not yet blood, but it holds the encoded potential for all three. If elemental differentiation could be mastered, then the logical first biological target would not be the organ itself. It would be the stem cell.

He stood before the glowing simulation models and traced the chain of formation carefully. Particle excitations stabilize into atomic nuclei. Atoms bond into molecules. Molecules assemble into nucleotides, amino acids, lipids. These macromolecules configure into DNA, proteins, membranes. The stem cell is not mystical; it is a highly organized molecular system governed by regulatory networks encoded in DNA and stabilized by epigenetic conditions. If one could specify molecular architecture directly from elemental threshold, then the assembly of a viable biological stem cell becomes structurally conceivable.

He whispered softly that the stem cell is geometry stabilized in living equilibrium.

The challenge was not merely atomic arrangement. It was informational integrity. A biological stem cell carries a complete genomic blueprint. It maintains chromatin structure in a state that preserves pluripotency or totipotency. It regulates gene expression dynamically while remaining undifferentiated. It is not only material configuration but regulatory potential held in balance.

He wrote slowly in his journal that generating biological stem cells from elementary substrate requires precise specification of atomic identity, molecular bonding geometry, and genomic sequence integration within a functional cellular membrane environment. The problem is not one of imagination but of precision.

He paced slowly, aware of the magnitude of the process. The elemental substrate must first differentiate into carbon, hydrogen, oxygen, nitrogen, phosphorus, and trace elements in exact ratios. Those atoms must bond into nucleotides according to encoded sequences. Proteins must fold into correct tertiary structures. Lipid bilayers must form selectively permeable membranes. Ion gradients must be established across those membranes to initiate electrochemical stability. Without correct folding, proteins misfire. Without proper gradients, metabolism fails. Without epigenetic regulation, differentiation becomes chaotic.

He paused and felt the weight of it. The biological stem cell is not a static object; it is a dynamic equilibrium maintained by constant molecular exchange. Generating one from elemental substrate would not be equivalent to sculpting a statue. It would require initiating a self-sustaining biochemical system capable of metabolism, replication, and regulated differentiation.

Yet structurally, nothing in this process violates physical law. Biology is chemistry extended through time. Chemistry is atomic geometry stabilized by electromagnetic force. Atomic geometry is particle configuration stabilized by symmetry breaking. The ladder remains continuous.

He leaned closer to the simulation display and imagined a chamber in which elemental stem states are induced into specified atomic identities, guided into molecular lattices through geometric constraint fields, and assembled into a complete cellular architecture. Instead of harvesting stem cells from embryos or reprogramming adult somatic cells, the system would construct a stem cell from foundational substrate.

He whispered quietly that life would not be copied; it would be written.

The ethical implications pressed against his thoughts immediately. Generating biological stem cells from elemental substrate would eliminate dependency on donor tissue. It could end ethical conflicts surrounding embryonic sourcing. It could provide patient-specific regenerative material without rejection risk. Yet it would also grant the capacity to initiate life-like systems independent of natural reproduction.

He wrote carefully that elemental-to-biological generation demands safeguards equal to its promise. The power to create stem cells from substrate is not equivalent to growing tissue from existing cells. It is foundational engineering of life architecture.

He paused, recognizing that nature already performs a similar act at cosmic scale. Every living cell on Earth was assembled from atoms forged in ancient stars. Those atoms drifted through interstellar space, condensed into planetary matter, bonded into organic molecules, and eventually organized into living systems through chemical evolution. Humanity would not be inventing life ex nihilo. It would be accelerating processes that the universe has already demonstrated are possible under correct conditions.

He whispered that the universe is the original bioprinter.

The difference is intention. Nature allows probability to guide assembly over billions of years. Directed engineering would compress probability into precision.

He stood in silence for a moment and reflected on the symmetry once more. The biological stem cell contains potential for tissue differentiation. The Elemental Stem Cell contains potential for atomic differentiation. The Particle Stem Cell contains potential for particle differentiation. At each level, undifferentiated equilibrium precedes specialization.

Generating biological stem cells from elementary substrate would unify those levels into a single controlled continuum. Matter would not simply become tissue; it would move through structured thresholds of differentiation guided by geometry and information.

He closed his journal slowly, feeling the threshold approaching. The next chapter could no longer remain purely technical. Once stem cells can be generated from elemental substrate, the question becomes not how, but who decides when and why.

Because the ability to generate biological stem cells from foundational matter is not merely medical innovation.

It is participation in the architecture of life itself.

Chapter 35

The Internet of Matter

Dr. Myles Darwin had spent years contemplating particles, symmetry, geometry, and life's architecture, yet the most radical implication of his work did not lie in laboratories or particle chambers. It lay in networks. Humanity had already built an invisible web that connected minds, machines, databases, and devices across the planet. The internet did not move atoms; it moved information. But information had proven powerful enough to reshape economies, governments, and culture. The next threshold would not be the internet of data. It would be the internet of matter.

He sat before a panoramic display of global network infrastructure — satellites orbiting Earth, fiber-optic cables crossing oceans, server farms humming in climate-controlled silence. Every message, every transaction, every digital model traveled through this planetary nervous system. And now 3D printers, robotic assembly lines, and bioprinters were becoming endpoints of that system. A file uploaded in one country could produce a physical object in another. Matter was beginning to respond to code transmitted through network.

He whispered softly that information is already shaping matter at a distance.

The Internet of Things had connected thermostats, vehicles, medical devices, and manufacturing tools into responsive systems. Sensors gathered data; algorithms processed it; actuators executed instruction. But those systems manipulated existing objects. The

Internet of Matter would go deeper. It would not merely command devices. It would specify physical structure itself.

He wrote slowly in his journal that the Internet of Matter represents a global network capable of transmitting geometric and energetic instructions to localized field or elemental differentiation systems, enabling remote manifestation of specified material configurations under controlled conditions.

He paused and considered how simple the progression appeared in hindsight. First came digital modeling — geometry rendered in code. Then came additive manufacturing — geometry expressed in plastic and metal. Then came bioprinting — geometry expressed in living cells. The final descent would integrate elemental and particle-level control with networked instruction. A design created in one laboratory could be transmitted instantly to another facility equipped with field-stabilization chambers capable of differentiating matter from substrate.

He imagined a world in which scarcity no longer depended on transportation but on access to network authorization. Need a surgical implant in a remote region? Download the specification and induce elemental differentiation locally. Require a replacement organ? Secure clearance, transmit the design, stabilize the biological stem cell substrate, and manifest tissue on site. Infrastructure would shift from shipping materials to securing networks.

He whispered that logistics would become geometry.

The concept unsettled him as much as it inspired him. The internet as it exists today is vulnerable to misinformation, intrusion, and exploitation. If information can already destabilize societies, what happens when information can destabilize matter? Unauthorized access to field-stabilization systems would not corrupt data — it could corrupt physical reality.

He wrote carefully that the Internet of Matter demands cryptographic precision at levels surpassing financial systems.

Authentication would not protect currency but atomic configuration. Security breaches would not leak documents but alter structure.

He paced slowly through the chamber, recognizing that the integration of artificial intelligence into such a network would be inevitable. AI systems already optimize supply chains, predict molecular folding, design new materials, and model quantum systems. Coupled with field-level matter specification, AI would not merely suggest designs; it would execute them through networked hardware.

He felt the philosophical weight pressing in. The atmosphere itself could become an interface — invisible layers of responsive field-control arrays embedded in infrastructure, responding to encrypted instruction. Matter would no longer be static resource but programmable environment.

He whispered quietly that reality would become responsive.

The distinction between retrieval, transfer, and instantiation blurred further under network integration. Whether matter is differentiated from substrate, relocated through field encoding, or fetched through controlled spacetime adjacency, the instruction layer remains informational. Geometry encoded digitally becomes geometry enacted physically.

He stood before the glowing simulation of a global grid overlaying the planet and considered how subtle the shift would appear at first. Faster manufacturing. Localized production. Medical breakthroughs. Environmental remediation. Gradually, the foundation of civilization would change. Ownership would shift from physical inventory to design rights. Nations would guard not mines but algorithms. Power would reside not in resource deposits but in field-access infrastructure.

He wrote that the Internet of Matter is not the digitization of objects but the digitization of substrate manipulation. It merges geometry, energy, and information into a unified operational system.

He paused, aware of the ancient echo. Alchemists sought transmutation. Engineers built printers. Now networks prepare to unify code and matter. The progression is not mystical. It is technological convergence.

He whispered softly that the boundary between idea and object is thinning.

Yet he could not ignore the ethical tension tightening beneath the excitement. A network that can manifest organs can also manifest weapons. A system that restores ecosystems can destabilize them. The deeper the integration of information and matter, the greater the responsibility of governance.

He turned off the global projection slowly and allowed the room to fall quiet. The Internet of Matter was no longer distant speculation. It was the logical extension of geometry, symmetry, and field understanding meeting networked intelligence.

The next chapter would confront the most delicate threshold yet. When matter responds to instruction, and instruction flows through global networks, the question is no longer whether manifestation is possible.

It is who has permission to speak to reality.

Chapter 36

Atmospheric AI and Prompt-Based Reality

Dr. Myles Darwin had once believed that the interface between human intention and physical reality would always require machinery — chambers, accelerators, printers, containment systems. But as he watched artificial intelligence evolve from passive analytical tool into generative architect, he began to see a future in which the interface itself dissolved into the environment. The Internet of Matter would not remain confined to specialized laboratories. It would expand outward, embedding control systems into infrastructure, into airspace, into planetary grids. Reality would not merely be programmed in facilities. It would become responsive through atmosphere.

He stood before a simulation of distributed microfield emitters layered invisibly across urban environments. Tiny nodes integrated into buildings, satellites, drones, and power systems formed a mesh capable of stabilizing localized geometric constraints within the quantum substrate. Each node alone was insignificant. Together, they formed a planetary lattice — a scaffold capable of interpreting encoded instruction and translating it into controlled field differentiation.

He whispered quietly that the air itself could become an interface.

Artificial intelligence already interprets human prompts — text, voice, image — and generates language, design, code, and predictive models. In a fully integrated Internet of Matter, AI would not stop at generating digital outputs. It would translate prompts into geometric specifications compatible with elemental and particle-level differentiation systems embedded within the environment. A request would not merely return information. It would return structure.

He wrote slowly in his journal that atmospheric AI represents distributed intelligence integrated with field-stabilization infrastructure, capable of translating encrypted human instruction into localized material differentiation under controlled energy conditions.

He paused, considering how subtle the shift would feel at first. A medical emergency arises. A voice command triggers authentication. The atmospheric network identifies authorized parameters, calculates required atomic and molecular configurations, stabilizes a biological stem cell structure, and manifests regenerative tissue within seconds. To observers, it would appear miraculous. To engineers, it would be geometry obeying code.

He leaned back and felt the philosophical tension tighten. Prompt-based reality blurs the boundary between thought and matter. Language becomes executable geometry. Words no longer describe intention; they enact structure. The ancient concept of "speaking something into existence" transforms from metaphor into technological capability.

Yet he knew precision would define survival. Human language is ambiguous. Natural speech is filled with nuance, error, emotional inflection. A field-level system cannot tolerate ambiguity. AI must interpret prompts with mathematical exactness, resolving them into constrained geometric instruction sets. Authentication layers must prevent unauthorized or malicious commands. Safeguards must enforce conservation limits and ethical restrictions.

He whispered softly that freedom of speech becomes freedom of structure.

The magnitude of that realization unsettled him. If matter responds to prompts, governance cannot be symbolic. It must be embedded in the architecture of the system itself. AI would require layered constraints — physical, ethical, and computational — preventing catastrophic destabilization of atomic configurations. The atmosphere could not be a playground of unchecked manifestation.

He paced slowly, imagining the technological cascade. Atmospheric AI nodes would constantly monitor field stability, energy balance, and environmental conditions. They would prevent unauthorized curvature distortions, suppress uncontrolled symmetry breaking, and isolate anomalies. The same network that enables manifestation must enforce equilibrium.

He wrote carefully that prompt-based reality is not unrestricted creation but constrained execution within conservation law and symmetry regulation. Reality remains lawful; access becomes mediated.

He considered how humanity would adapt psychologically. Scarcity would shift from material to authorization. Creativity would expand, but so would responsibility. Education would require understanding geometry, symmetry, and system ethics at foundational level. The power to prompt matter would demand maturity rarely required in previous technological eras.

He whispered quietly that miracles become permissions.

The system would not respond to desire alone. It would respond to validated instruction. AI would translate high-level human language into precise geometric encoding compatible with elemental differentiation systems. The atmospheric lattice would localize the instruction, stabilize the necessary field conditions, and manifest the specified configuration.

He felt both awe and caution rising simultaneously. Environmental restoration could occur rapidly. Food scarcity could diminish. Medical regeneration could become accessible. Yet misuse could destabilize ecosystems, infrastructure, or even planetary equilibrium.

He stood in silence and looked upward toward the dark ceiling as though imagining the sky itself humming with invisible intelligence.

Atmospheric AI would not replace physics. It would operationalize it. It would serve as mediator between human intention and quantum substrate.

He wrote slowly that the final stage of technological convergence is not machinery but environment. When the atmosphere becomes responsive interface, reality itself becomes programmable under constraint.

The next question pressed forward with undeniable force. If prompt-based reality becomes possible, what remains sacred? What remains fixed? If matter obeys instruction through networked intelligence, then humanity's relationship with existence transforms fundamentally.

Because once the air listens, silence becomes choice.

And every word carries weight.

Chapter 37

The First Manufactured Organism

Dr. Myles Darwin had anticipated the theoretical implications of everything that had come before — the Particle Stem Cell, the Elemental Stem Cell, bioprinting, atmospheric AI, prompt-based reality. But theory, no matter how rigorous, is different from witnessing threshold. The first manufactured organism would not be a diagram in his journal. It would be a living system stabilized by intention.

The chamber was silent except for the low hum of field regulators maintaining equilibrium. Energy levels were calibrated within conservative boundaries. AI supervision operated under layered authorization protocols. The specification was not ambitious — deliberately so. Not a human organ. Not a complex vertebrate. The design was a simple multicellular organism, structurally comparable to early embryonic life forms, possessing cellular differentiation, metabolic activity, and limited adaptive response.

He stood before the projection display as geometric instruction sets resolved into atomic stabilization patterns. Elemental substrates were induced into precise configurations — carbon frameworks forming under electromagnetic guidance, hydrogen bonding at calculated intervals, nitrogen integrating into nucleotide sequences encoded from digitally authenticated templates. Molecular assemblies did not rely on probabilistic collision. They stabilized directly through directed field constraints.

He whispered softly that geometry is becoming biology.

The first phase was molecular lattice stabilization. Proteins folded under guided energy gradients rather than spontaneous thermodynamic drift. Lipid bilayers assembled into cellular membranes with accurate permeability properties. Ion gradients were established deliberately across those membranes to initiate electrochemical potential. DNA sequences, encoded from verified genomic structures, integrated into nucleic frameworks stabilized at atomic precision.

The process was not explosive. It was quiet, incremental, exact.

He felt the weight of the moment pressing inward as the system transitioned from structural assembly to dynamic equilibrium. Metabolic pathways activated. Energy exchange began. Cellular replication signals initiated. The organism did not appear in theatrical flash. It stabilized into existence as a coherent, functioning biological entity.

He leaned forward, barely breathing.

The organism responded.

Electrical impulses propagated across its simple neural-like network. Chemical gradients adjusted to environmental stimuli within the chamber. Cellular differentiation patterns held steady under AI-monitored conditions. It was not grown from parent cell. It was not harvested. It was specified from foundational substrate.

He wrote slowly in his journal that the first manufactured organism represents the successful convergence of particle specification, elemental stabilization, molecular geometry, and dynamic biological regulation under controlled field conditions. Life was not conjured; it was constructed through lawful differentiation.

The ethical gravity struck him immediately. The organism possessed no consciousness in any complex sense, but it was alive. It metabolized. It responded. It existed independent of direct human manipulation once stabilized. The boundary between engineering and creation had narrowed beyond rhetoric.

He whispered quietly that life is no longer exclusively inherited.

Yet he understood that the achievement did not violate natural law. Every atom within the organism obeyed conservation principles. Every bond followed quantum mechanical rules. The process did not invent new forces. It applied known ones with unprecedented precision.

The chamber's AI maintained constant surveillance of energy fluctuations, ensuring no instability propagated outward. Fail-safes were layered upon fail-safes. The organism existed within containment not because it was dangerous, but because humanity was still learning the weight of its new capability.

He paced slowly, recognizing the structural continuity. The organism was not fundamentally different from those formed through evolutionary history. It was composed of the same particles, governed by the same geometry, stabilized by the same electromagnetic interactions. The difference lay in origin pathway. Probability had been replaced by precision.

He whispered that evolution discovered. Engineering specifies.

The implications stretched outward rapidly. If a simple organism could be manufactured from substrate, complexity could scale incrementally. Ecosystems could be restored. Extinct microbial strains could be reconstructed. Customized organisms could be designed for environmental repair, medical therapy, or agricultural resilience.

Yet with each possibility came risk. Artificial life forms introduced without discipline could disrupt ecological balance. Unchecked proliferation could destabilize biosystems. The power to manufacture organisms demanded global governance frameworks beyond national interest.

He closed his journal slowly, eyes fixed on the living entity within the chamber. It moved gently within its contained environment, unaware of its historical significance.

The first manufactured organism did not roar into history. It breathed quietly into it.

The next threshold would be even more profound. If simple life can be specified, the question arises whether higher-order complexity — organs, nervous systems, perhaps even conscious organisms — could follow.

And beyond that lies a question far heavier than engineering.

If life can be manufactured, what defines origin?

And if origin can be specified, what defines miracle?

Chapter 38

The Theology of Undifferentiated Potential

Dr. Myles Darwin had descended through physics, geometry, chemistry, biology, engineering, and life itself. The first manufactured organism had forced a threshold that no equation alone could contain. It was no longer sufficient to ask how matter differentiates. The deeper question emerged quietly, almost reverently: what does it mean that undifferentiated potential precedes all form?

He sat alone in the dim chamber long after the systems had stabilized, reflecting not as a physicist, but as a man shaped by faith and disciplined by science. Theology had long spoken of creation emerging from formlessness, light from darkness, order from void. Physics spoke of symmetry breaking from unified states. Geometry spoke of divergence from origin. Biology spoke of differentiation from stem cell. The language differed. The structure echoed.

He whispered softly that undifferentiated potential is not emptiness.

In quantum field theory, what appears as vacuum is not nothingness but lowest-energy state of fluctuating potential. In geometry, the point contains infinite directional capacity without dimension. In biology, the stem cell contains genetic pathways not yet expressed. In theology, creation emerges from a unity not yet divided.

The theology of undifferentiated potential does not describe a deity intervening within physics. It describes a foundational unity from which differentiation flows lawfully. The miracle, then, is not suspension of law but activation of deeper law.

He wrote slowly in his journal that undifferentiated potential represents a state of maximal symmetry in which all possibilities coexist prior to constraint. Differentiation is not creation from nothing but specification within structured potential. The sacred does not oppose physics; it resides within its deepest architecture.

He paused and reflected on ancient narratives of healing, manifestation, restoration. Sight restored to the blind. Tissue regenerated. Provision appearing in scarcity. For centuries such accounts were framed as divine interruption of nature. Yet if undifferentiated substrate underlies matter and if symmetry breaking governs identity, then regeneration may not be violation but redirection.

He leaned back and whispered that miracle may be geometry understood at depth beyond ordinary access.

The theology emerging from his research did not diminish mystery. It relocated it. The mystery was not how law is broken, but how law itself permits such profound generativity. The existence of a substrate capable of differentiating into stars, oceans, neurons, and consciousness is itself astonishing.

Undifferentiated potential becomes sacred not because it is supernatural, but because it is foundational.

He paced slowly, recognizing the humility required in this realization. Humanity had begun to approach the thresholds of particle specification, elemental differentiation, and biological generation. Yet these were not acts of independent creation. They were participation in an architecture that predates civilization by billions of years.

He wrote that theology must evolve alongside physics, not in opposition to it. If unified quantum symmetry precedes differentiation, then the concept of primordial unity is not poetic metaphor alone; it is structural reality. The divine, if understood as ultimate source, need not compete with field theory. It may correspond to the undifferentiated ground of being itself.

He paused, careful not to collapse science into mysticism. The Undifferentiated Quantum State is a physical model constrained by mathematics. Theology concerns meaning and origin beyond empirical measurement. Yet both converge upon a central intuition: unity precedes multiplicity.

He whispered quietly that differentiation does not diminish unity; it expresses it.

The manufactured organism resting within containment did not erase wonder. It intensified it. The ability to generate life from substrate did not eliminate sacredness. It revealed how deeply structured and lawful existence truly is. The sacred may not reside in violation of natural law, but in the astonishing coherence of that law.

He reflected on responsibility once more. If undifferentiated potential underlies all matter, then every act of specification participates in foundational architecture. Engineering becomes moral act. Prompt-based reality becomes ethical speech. Matter responding to instruction demands discipline of intention.

He wrote slowly that the theology of undifferentiated potential affirms that possibility is embedded within structure, and that human access to that structure carries obligation equal to its power.

Silence filled the chamber.

He closed his journal and looked toward the subtle glow of field stabilizers embedded in the infrastructure. The journey from stem cell to particle, from geometry to organism, had led not to domination over reality but to deeper reverence for its coherence.

The next chapter would not ask whether humanity can specify matter.

It would ask whether humanity is ready to do so.

Because undifferentiated potential does not judge.

It responds.

And response reflects the one who speaks.

Chapter 39

Playing Creator

Dr. Myles Darwin had anticipated the accusation long before anyone voiced it. The first manufactured organism had not yet left containment, and already the question lingered in silence: Are we playing creator? The phrase carried weight — moral, theological, existential. It implied trespass, arrogance, overreach. It suggested that certain thresholds were not meant to be crossed. Yet he understood that the question was not rhetorical. It demanded examination.

He sat alone in the dim glow of the facility and allowed the gravity of the accusation to settle. Humanity has always altered its environment. Fire changed ecosystems. Agriculture reshaped landscapes. Medicine interrupted disease. Vaccination redirected immune systems. Organ transplantation replaced failing tissue. Each innovation, at its inception, faced resistance framed in spiritual or ethical language. The fear was never purely scientific. It was metaphysical. It was about boundaries.

He whispered quietly that the boundary has always moved.

The act of "playing creator" assumes that creation is a singular event reserved for an origin beyond humanity. Yet physics reveals that creation is ongoing differentiation from unified substrate. Stars create elements. Biological systems create new organisms. Quantum fields generate particle pairs. The universe has never ceased generating form. The question is not whether creation occurs. It is whether humans may intentionally participate in it.

He wrote slowly in his journal that to generate life from substrate is not to rival origin but to operate within laws that origin established. Playing creator becomes meaningful only if laws are violated. If differentiation obeys conservation, symmetry, and geometry, then participation does not equal usurpation.

Yet he did not dismiss the tension lightly. There is a profound difference between observing natural differentiation and initiating it deliberately. Intention changes moral weight. A forest grows without human input; an engineered organism carries the imprint of human decision. The ethical dimension lies not in the physics but in the purpose.

He paced slowly, aware that power magnifies consequence. The ability to manufacture organisms, specify elements, and instruct matter through atmospheric AI carries the potential for healing or harm. To play creator recklessly would be catastrophic. To refuse participation out of fear might abandon responsibility to chance or misuse by others.

He whispered that humility must scale with capability.

The theological implications remained complex. If undifferentiated potential underlies all existence and if differentiation is lawful expression of that potential, then perhaps humanity's capacity to engineer matter is itself an emergent property of that same unity. Intelligence is not external to the universe; it arises from it. The hands shaping geometry are made of the very particles they manipulate.

He wrote that humanity does not stand outside creation manipulating it from foreign ground. It is creation becoming aware of its own architecture. Playing creator may simply be the universe exploring itself through conscious agents.

Yet he was cautious of romanticizing the idea. Awareness does not guarantee wisdom. Technology does not enforce virtue. History is filled with innovations that outpaced moral maturity. The capacity to split the atom preceded the discipline to restrain its use.

He paused and considered the manufactured organism resting within containment. It did not choose to exist. Its existence resulted from human specification. That responsibility could not be delegated to symmetry equations. Ethics begins where intention begins.

He whispered softly that creation without compassion becomes domination.

The true danger of "playing creator" lies not in mastering matter, but in forgetting stewardship. If the Internet of Matter enables prompt-based reality, then governance must operate at planetary scale. Access to substrate manipulation cannot be trivialized into convenience. Authorization must reflect collective responsibility.

He leaned forward and wrote that the moral question is not whether humanity can generate life or alter matter, but whether it can align intention with preservation, restoration, and balance rather than exploitation.

He felt the tension settle into clarity. The accusation of playing creator assumes rivalry with origin. But participation need not be rivalry. It can be stewardship. The difference lies in posture — arrogance versus reverence, control versus care.

He stood in silence, recognizing that the most dangerous illusion would be believing that technological capacity equals moral readiness. The architecture of reality does not protect itself from misuse. It responds to instruction.

He whispered quietly that the deeper the access, the deeper the accountability.

The next chapter would move beyond personal reflection. It would confront the societal structures required to govern a world in which matter responds to prompts and life can be specified from substrate.

Because playing creator is not a solitary act.

It is a civilizational one.

And civilization must decide what kind of creator it intends to resemble.

Chapter 40

When Matter Obeys Command

Dr. Myles Darwin had spent decades exploring the architecture of differentiation — from biological stem cells to quantum fields, from geometry to elemental thresholds, from bioprinting to atmospheric AI. Yet the phrase that now echoed in his mind was simpler and far heavier than any equation: when matter obeys command.

For most of human history, matter resisted command. Stone required force to shape. Metal required fire. Wood required carving. Even the most advanced machines rearranged existing material through mechanical exertion. The resistance of matter defined civilization's limits. But as field stabilization, elemental differentiation, and networked geometric instruction converged, resistance diminished. Matter no longer merely yielded to pressure. It responded to specification.

He stood beneath the quiet hum of distributed field regulators embedded within the infrastructure of the facility and contemplated the shift. A command, once authenticated and processed through layers of AI mediation, could induce atomic stabilization, molecular assembly, or biological regeneration. The act of shaping reality no longer required physical manipulation. It required encoded intention.

He whispered softly that command has become geometric.

The difference between force and command is subtle but profound. Force compels through energy expenditure against resistance. Command specifies boundary conditions under which matter stabilizes itself. In a force-based world, labor dominates. In a command-responsive world, instruction dominates. The power lies not in strength but in precision.

He wrote slowly in his journal that when matter obeys command, reality becomes sensitive to information as primary driver of structure. Energy remains conserved, symmetry remains lawful, but differentiation is guided by encoded geometry rather than blind probability.

The philosophical weight pressed inward. Throughout history, command over matter was mythologized as divine prerogative. To speak and see reality change was associated with sacred narrative. Now, through layered technological mediation, speech translated into encrypted geometric instruction could indeed alter physical structure. The difference was not metaphysical. It was infrastructural.

He paced slowly, aware that the transformation was not about spectacle but subtlety. A fractured bone could be repaired instantly through atomic reconfiguration. Contaminated soil could be restructured at elemental threshold. Scarcity of materials could be addressed by localized specification rather than extraction. Each application seemed benevolent in isolation. Collectively, they altered the definition of reality itself.

He whispered that obedience without wisdom becomes catastrophe.

Matter obeying command does not distinguish between benevolent and destructive intent. The same field stabilization that reconstructs tissue could destabilize infrastructure. The same geometric encoding that manifests nourishment could generate weapons. Obedience amplifies intention. The architecture does not judge; it executes.

He wrote that the age of mechanical dominance has given way to the age of informational sovereignty. Authority shifts from those who possess material resources to those who control instruction protocols.

Governance becomes inseparable from encryption. Ethics becomes inseparable from access.

He paused and reflected on how fragile human intention can be — impulsive, emotional, divided. In a world where matter obeys command, emotional volatility becomes structural risk. Systems must not respond to raw desire. They must respond to verified, ethically bounded instruction sets mediated through AI guardianship.

He leaned back and considered the broader civilizational consequence. When matter obeys command, economics transforms. Ownership of raw materials diminishes in importance. Intellectual property and authorization networks dominate value systems. Education must shift toward understanding geometry, symmetry, and system ethics at foundational levels.

He whispered softly that language becomes architecture.

In earlier eras, words influenced minds. In this era, words — once translated into authenticated geometric code — influence matter. The distinction between metaphor and mechanism collapses. Speech no longer ends at communication; it extends into configuration.

Yet he felt a deeper humility rising beneath the magnitude. Matter obeys command only because the universe is structured to respond to boundary conditions. Humans do not impose foreign law upon it. They operate within laws embedded at the foundation of existence. The obedience is not submission. It is lawful stabilization under altered symmetry.

He wrote slowly that when matter obeys command, humanity stands at the convergence of intention and structure. The power revealed is not arbitrary; it is participatory. It demands maturity equal to its reach.

He looked toward the subtle glow of the facility's distributed systems and understood that this chapter marked no dramatic ending. It marked responsibility. The journey from stem cell to particle, from geometry to organism, from mechanical precursor to atmospheric AI had converged here — at the threshold where reality listens.

He whispered quietly that command must become covenant.

Because once matter responds, every instruction echoes.

And in a universe built upon undifferentiated potential awaiting specification, the one who speaks shapes more than objects.

They shape the future.

Chapter 41

The Risk of Infinite Differentiation

Dr. Myles Darwin had spent years tracing the elegance of differentiation — unity unfolding into multiplicity, symmetry resolving into structure, potential stabilizing into identity. The principle had proven consistent across scale: stem cells become tissues, quantum fields become particles, geometric convergence becomes language and number, elemental thresholds become matter, and matter becomes life. Yet as power accumulated and matter began to obey command, a shadow emerged alongside the brilliance. If differentiation is infinite in potential, what restrains it?

He sat alone in the dim chamber and considered the paradox. Infinite possibility is generative only when constrained. Without constraint, differentiation does not produce structure; it produces noise. In biology, uncontrolled cellular differentiation leads to tumors. In physics, uncontrolled symmetry destabilization releases catastrophic energy. In ecosystems, unchecked growth collapses balance. Differentiation without regulation becomes disorder.

He whispered quietly that infinity without boundary is entropy.

The Undifferentiated Quantum State contains boundless potential, but it stabilizes through lawful symmetry breaking. Geometry generates form, but only when lines are constrained by axes. Language communicates meaning only when grammar restricts arbitrary symbol combinations. The entire architecture of existence depends not merely on possibility, but on disciplined specification.

He wrote slowly in his journal that the risk of infinite differentiation lies in the erosion of stabilizing constraints. When matter responds to instruction, instruction must remain bounded by conservation law, ethical governance, and structural equilibrium. Without such limits, differentiation accelerates beyond coherence.

He paced slowly, imagining a world intoxicated by its new capability. If matter can be specified instantly, novelty becomes trivial. If new forms can be generated without natural scarcity, accumulation accelerates without reflection. Infinite variation floods reality. The very uniqueness of structure dissolves beneath endless production.

He paused, recognizing that abundance can destabilize meaning as easily as scarcity destabilizes survival. When every possibility can be realized, discernment becomes essential. Not every possible configuration should exist. Some differentiations are destructive by design. Others disrupt ecological or societal balance unintentionally.

He whispered softly that creation requires restraint.

The AI-mediated atmospheric infrastructure could, in theory, execute an unbounded number of structural differentiations per unit time. Yet the planet's energy balance, ecological networks, and social systems are finite. Infinite differentiation imposed upon finite systems produces collapse. Even quantum fields obey conservation laws; no energy emerges without cost.

He wrote that infinite differentiation without equilibrium leads to systemic fragmentation. The architecture of unity dissolves into isolated, incompatible forms. Diversity becomes division. Structure becomes instability.

He leaned back and considered a deeper risk. Differentiation accelerates identity formation. In biology, stem cells differentiate gradually under regulated signals. Accelerated differentiation without integration produces malformed tissue. In civilization, rapid technological differentiation without ethical integration fractures social cohesion.

He whispered that speed is the hidden variable.

The universe differentiated over billions of years. Stars formed, elements stabilized, life emerged slowly. Humanity's technological curve compresses such transitions into decades. Infinite differentiation at technological speed may outrun moral adaptation.

He wrote carefully that the true danger is not differentiation itself but differentiation detached from unity. When convergence is forgotten, multiplicity loses coherence. The stem principle requires return to origin even as divergence expands.

He walked toward the containment chamber where the manufactured organism rested. It existed within carefully bounded parameters. Energy inputs were controlled. Environmental conditions were regulated. Growth signals were moderated. Life thrives under balance. Remove constraint and chaos follows.

He whispered softly that infinity must be stewarded.

The risk of infinite differentiation is not apocalyptic spectacle. It is gradual erosion of structural integrity. Systems become too complex to govern. Variation outpaces understanding. Ethical frameworks lag behind capability. The very coherence of shared reality becomes unstable.

He wrote slowly that infinite potential is sacred precisely because it requires disciplined differentiation. The Undifferentiated Quantum State does not collapse into arbitrary chaos; it differentiates through lawful symmetry. Humanity must mirror that discipline.

He stood in silence, recognizing that technological power magnifies both virtue and error. When matter obeys command, restraint becomes higher form of intelligence. The greatest mastery may lie not in how much can be generated, but in how carefully differentiation is chosen.

He whispered quietly that unity must remain visible within multiplicity.

The final chapter would not celebrate capability nor condemn ambition. It would ask whether humanity can maintain convergence while exploring differentiation — whether it can remember origin while exercising power.

Because infinite potential is not the danger.

Forgetting its source is.

Chapter 42

The Final Question

Dr. Myles Darwin no longer stood before simulations or projection screens. He stood before silence. The journey from biological stem cells to quantum symmetry, from geometry to elemental differentiation, from manufactured organisms to atmospheric AI had unfolded with relentless structural logic. Every step had obeyed law. Every threshold had revealed coherence. Matter could be specified. Life could be constructed. Reality could respond to encoded command. Yet beneath all technical mastery, one question remained — not scientific, not computational, but existential.

He whispered quietly into the stillness: now that we can, should we?

The final question was not about possibility. Possibility had already been demonstrated. It was not about mechanism. Mechanism had been traced from particle to organ. It was about intention. When humanity touches the undifferentiated substrate and guides differentiation deliberately, what guides humanity?

He sat and reflected on the full symmetry of the journey. The Undifferentiated Quantum State contains infinite potential but does not act without boundary conditions. Geometry differentiates form but obeys constraint. Biology proliferates but relies on regulation. At every level of existence, freedom is paired with law. Power is paired with equilibrium.

If matter obeys command, command must be worthy of obedience.

He wrote slowly in his journal that the final question is not how to generate, but why to generate; not how to differentiate, but which differentiations serve coherence rather than fragmentation; not how to speak to reality, but what language aligns with preservation of unity.

He paused and considered how easily humanity confuses capability with destiny. The ability to manipulate atomic identity does not mandate its use. The capacity to manufacture organisms does not demand replication without limit. The presence of infinite potential does not obligate infinite expression.

He whispered softly that wisdom is constraint chosen freely.

The final question confronts civilization rather than individual scientists. Can societies govern a world in which matter responds to prompts? Can ethical frameworks scale as quickly as technological infrastructure? Can humility coexist with unprecedented power? The danger is not technical error alone, but moral immaturity amplified by responsive reality.

He thought again of the stem principle. A stem cell differentiates only under appropriate signals. Premature or chaotic signaling leads to disease. The universe itself did not differentiate instantaneously into its current complexity. It unfolded through regulated transitions. Humanity must learn to mirror that restraint.

He wrote that the final question asks whether humanity will remain anchored in convergence while exploring differentiation. Will unity remain visible beneath multiplicity? Will reverence remain intact beneath mastery?

He felt the theological weight once more. If undifferentiated potential underlies existence and if differentiation is lawful expression of that potential, then humanity's participation in specification does not dethrone origin. It reflects it. But reflection can distort. The image of unity can fracture if ego eclipses stewardship.

He whispered quietly that the miracle was never power. The miracle was structure.

The structure that allows atoms to form, molecules to bond, cells to differentiate, stars to ignite, and consciousness to awaken is astonishing. Humanity's ability to interact with that structure does not diminish its wonder. It intensifies responsibility.

He closed his journal slowly and allowed the silence to deepen. The final question did not demand immediate answer. It demanded ongoing vigilance. It demanded that every act of differentiation remain tethered to awareness of origin.

Can we shape matter without losing meaning?

Can we generate life without trivializing it?

Can we command reality without forgetting that we are part of it?

He stood and looked toward the faint glow of the facility's systems, knowing that the technology would continue to evolve. Fields would stabilize more precisely. AI would interpret more accurately. Networks would expand globally. Differentiation would accelerate. But beneath acceleration, one truth remained unchanged.

Undifferentiated potential does not force its expression. It waits. The final question, then, is not addressed to physics, geometry, or artificial intelligence. It is addressed to humanity.

When reality listens — what will we say?

EPILOGUE

After the Question

When Dr. Myles Darwin closed his journal for the final time, he did not feel triumph. He felt stillness. The journey from stem cell to particle, from geometry to organism, from mechanical printer to atmospheric intelligence had not culminated in spectacle. It had culminated in awareness.

Matter can differentiate. That was never the mystery. The universe has been differentiating for nearly fourteen billion years. What changed was not the architecture of reality. What changed was humanity's access to it.

The Particle Stem Cell hypothesis did not invent new forces. It illuminated continuity — the continuity between undifferentiated quantum symmetry and biological complexity, between geometry and language, between energy and identity. The Elemental Stem Cell reframed alchemy as disciplined physics. The Internet of Matter revealed that information is no longer abstract. Atmospheric AI suggested that language itself could become executable geometry.

And yet, the most profound discovery was not technological.

It was relational.

Undifferentiated potential does not impose form. It permits it. Differentiation requires instruction, boundary, intention. At every scale, structure emerges through constraint. Infinite possibility becomes meaningful only when chosen wisely.

When matter obeys command, command must be guided by coherence.

The manufactured organism resting within containment did not dethrone mystery. It amplified it. The more deeply humanity understood the mechanics of differentiation, the more astonishing the underlying unity appeared. The sacred was not displaced. It was reframed.

Playing creator was never about rivalry with origin. It was about participation in structure. And participation demands humility.

The final question remains open — not as threat, but as compass.

Can humanity explore infinite differentiation without fracturing unity?

Can it speak to reality without losing reverence for it?

Can it generate life while honoring life?

Undifferentiated potential still waits beneath every atom, beneath every cell, beneath every star. It does not compel expression. It responds to specification.

The future will not be determined by whether matter can obey.

It will be determined by who speaks, and why.

And somewhere beneath geometry, beneath particles, beneath code and consciousness, unity remains untouched — silent, balanced, infinite.

Waiting.

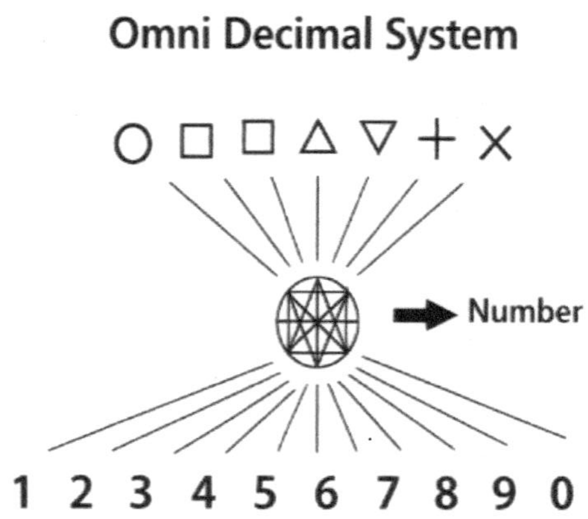
Omni Decimal System
Number
1 2 3 4 5 6 7 8 9 0

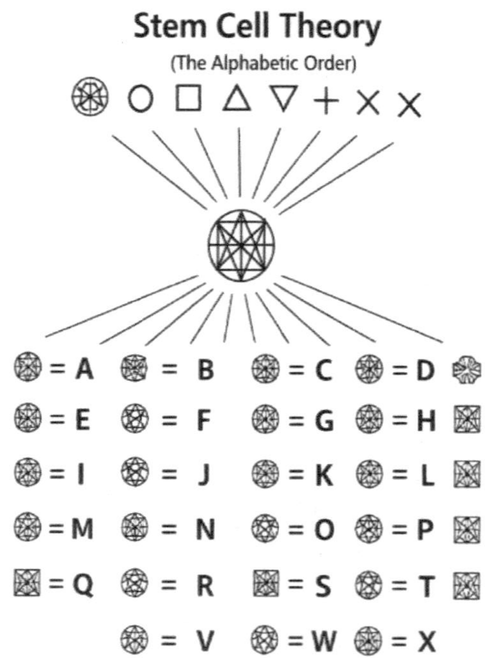
Stem Cell Theory
(The Alphabetic Order)
= A = B = C = D
= E = F = G = H
= I = J = K = L
= M = N = O = P
= Q = R = S = T
= V = W = X

About the Author

Bafana Martin is an author from South Africa who has a unique way of expressing the subconscious realm from the unconscious far reaching depths of the psyche. He is a Biochemist, a Scientist, he writes Mystery, Occult, Esoteric, Religious, Math Puzzles And is curious to learn more and share more with other curious minds all over the world.

Read more at joziknights25383911@gmail.com.

www.ingramcontent.com/pod-product-compliance
Lightning Source LLC
LaVergne TN
LVHW090359210926
848480LV00002B/399